FAT

IS OUR

FRIEND

How I found out that eating fat doesn't make you fat,
that saturated fat keeps you healthier...
and that Katy could lose 20 kilos without feeling hungry

Sammy Pepys

....the reluctant nutritionist

Fat is our Friend
First Edition published 2016 by
2QT Limited (Publishing)
Settle, North Yorkshire BD24 9RH United Kingdom

The author has his own website: www.fatisourfriend.com
Cover Design by Charlotte Mouncey
www.bookstyle.co.uk
Cover image supplied by istockphoto.com

Printed in Great Britain by
Lightning Source

A CIP catalogue record for this book is available
from the British Library
ISBN - 978-1-910077-81-8

Disclaimer

The information in this book tells the true story of Katy and others who have benefited from following the general guidelines outlined in these chapters. It is intended as a helpful guide to those of you interested in a healthy lifestyle, those of you who want to lose weight and those wanting to find greater energy to deal with life's many adventures. That being said, the book is not in any way a substitute for medical advice on your specific circumstances. Please consult your General Practitioner before changing, stopping or starting any medical treatment or new dietary regime.

A note on footnotes and web-links

While this book is not conceived as, nor does it purport to be, a scientific textbook, care has been taken to provide accurate references for those readers wishing to dig deeper into the many subjects covered. For your convenience and because Internet references can change from time to time, you will find a complete list of all links at the 'Fat is our Friend' website: www.fatisourfriend.com. This will also provide me with the opportunity to regularly monitor them for accuracy and add updated material when appropriate. For up-to-date information, you can also follow me on Twitter at #fatisourfriend, or use the hashtag #lchf for more general information on this subject from a mix of contributors.

Acknowledgements

Writing this would not have been possible without the love, support, patience and dietary adventurism of my wife Anne, my sons Oliver and Alexander, my daughter Rebecca and my nephew Lali, each of whom has bravely eaten their way through a number of dishes that were certainly not on the table a few years back. Others who have given feedback, contributed, cooked and provided rich food for thought include Anni, Graham, Elise, Pascal, Kerry, Tricia, Pierre, Annick, Katherine, Jeanne, Terry, Rob, Lynne, Steve, Karen and many others – my great appreciation goes out to all of you.

Special thanks go to Nella, who gave me the confidence to make this story much more of a personal journey rather than another textbook on the subject of diets and losing weight. I would also like to thank my brother Val as the first person generous enough to read through the whole manuscript and give helpful, critical and above all useful feedback and input. My editor Karen took this to the next level and worked painstakingly to make the book more coherent and flow logically. Any mistakes you may still find or observe are of my own doing and not down to my wonderful helpers.

Most importantly, I'd like to thank and congratulate Catherine (aka Katy) for having the courage and conviction to have one more go at healthy eating and, in so doing, avoiding the surgeon's knife. Without your faith and willpower, our little family world would be very different today.

Contents

PART 1

SETTING THE SCENE

Introduction

Why on earth should you read a book about healthy eating and dieting written by someone with no formal nutrition training? The answer is surprisingly simple. When I set out to discover the best ways for me and my immediate family not only to lose weight but to eat healthily, there was no ready answer; I discovered countless contradictions. The so-called experts – be they nutritionists, dieticians, doctors, medical researchers or the representatives of health organisations like the NHS in Britain or the American Heart Association in the US – only added to my confusion. I guess my problem is that I've never liked being simply told what to do. I'm still like one of those annoying four-year-olds who continually asks 'Why … ?' just because I need explanations; it's in my nature. And yet the many differing answers that I received to the simplest of questions, such as: 'What represents a balanced diet?' (especially when followed up with the question: '… and why is that?') just added to my initial confusion.

Because of all the contradictions and the lack of reasoned answers, I have spent much of the last three years reading books and scientific papers as well as talking to numerous 'experts' in an attempt to try and form an evidence-based, considered opinion. Whether or not you agree with my findings is, of course, up to you, but in one thing I am clear. You will find no more authoritative advice on the subject of healthy eating and diet because there are literally hundreds of different views out there. Even the PhDs cannot agree – in fact, some of them get involved in bitter in-fighting about each other's pet dietary theories.

In this book, I try to combine common sense with scientific facts. Where the facts have not been clearly established, I have used my best judgement. Simple as that. And yes, there has been a personal reason for this nutritional voyage of discovery. I find myself increasingly surrounded by people complaining of allergies or developing medical conditions such as diabetes – even becoming obese. Some strange sense of duty got me working with my sister-in-law to try and avoid the fitting of a gastric band. She had become obese over the years and needed to lose at least 10 kilos (for starters). Other diets had failed her. Not being the skinniest of men myself, I decided to join her in our jointly discovered regime to kick this journey off. I refused to allow short cuts such as protein shakes or dramatic reductions in calorie intake, though. We worked through a diet routine which, in essence, we could both follow for the long haul – but more of that later. As to the gluten- and lactose-troubled members of my family, we are working steadily through it. Lactose sensitivity is down. The gluten-free part appears more likely to be wheat intolerance, so we are working on that and discovering old forms of wheat such as einkorn to get us through (special thanks to Dr William Davis). As for my two picky eaters (a son and a niece) – well, they are learning to chop up their veggies so small before mixing them with meat in their home-made bolognaise sauce that even they can get a balanced meal. Whoops – did I say 'balanced'?!

This book is presented to you in eight main sections. After explaining how I got involved in the first place and talking through some of the unexpected facts discovered along the way (Part 1), I introduce Katy (Part 2), talk you through her healthy dietary approach (Part 3) and follow this up with important supporting evidence that I collected in the twin towns of Roseto (Part 4). My greatest learning experience, in many ways, was when I came to understand why counting calories is both misguided and doomed to failure; the next section (Part 5) is dedicated to that topic. Then, for those of you who want to dig deeper or just maybe are getting a little obsessed (as indeed I was), there's a section on food and digestion (Part 6). This reviews what we eat and how we go about digesting it – with a particular emphasis on fats and oils. Following this is a brief summary of the book so far (Part 7). If you'd like to read a more detailed analysis of my investigation focusing on the small township of Roseto in Pennsylvania (Part 8), you will find additional reasoning as to why I ended up favouring certain specific aspects of the so-called Mediterranean diet.

When it came to fats and oils, I came to the conclusion that a little more butter or lard in your cooking probably beats out olive oil – which still sounds a bit controversial to my ears today. Using as much olive oil as we like to in our cooking today is a relatively recent thing even for the French, the Italians and other aficionados of the favoured Mediterranean cuisine. Depending on your geographic location, natural saturated fats such as coconut oil, butter and lard have been used in cooking for millennia. But one thing is clear: the government subsidies which have encouraged the production of corn, soy, sunflower and all the other industrially produced seed oils have not made us healthier. Probably quite the opposite.

Do the so-called experts agree?

While I appreciate that in every scientific field there is a certain amount of learning by doing, and also that theories get further developed and updated over the years, there can surely be no other field containing so many diverse opinions as the area of nutrition – and no other field with such poor supporting research data. Fundamental 'truths' – such as the idea that higher levels of cholesterol are bad for you or that eating saturated fat causes heart disease – turn out to be incorrect or (at best) to be supported by dubious statistical correlation rather than scientific analysis.

When the experts do agree, semantics often hides their underlying disagreement. Junk food is bad for you – well, most of them would sign up for that. Yet, when asked for their definition of junk food, big differences appear. The reasons they give for why this junk food is not good for you also vary greatly.

Then we return to the whole balanced diet thing. The experts agree (again) that we should all be eating a balanced diet, but their definitions are often miles apart. 'Five a day' is one of the UK's healthy slogans. You'll find posters in schools and in doctors' waiting rooms around the country, rather like you used to see the American food pyramid poster in the United States – until it was changed, proven misleading and finally scrapped in 2010. 'Your 5 A DAY forms part of a healthy, balanced diet, and getting it is easier than you think,' says the NHS website.[1] But, as well as disagreeing on the content of a balanced diet, the experts are also in dispute over whether fruit and canned goods or ready-made soups are as good for you as fresh vegetables. Just like cans of baked beans in sweet tomato sauce, they all contribute to supporting your supposedly healthy eating habits as you count down towards your 'five a day'. An anomaly is nuts, which in their many forms were a staple food for our ancient

---

1   NHS, 2015 (1).

ancestors. Today, they are considered to have too high a fat content to be recommended as part of your 'five a day' diet. Sounds a bit wacky to me!

Fibre. Everyone knows we should be getting more fibre in our diets. After all, 'wholemeal bread is good for you'. Surely, most people agree with that statement? Not so, say members of the growing paleo diet community, who believe that our genes are still much better adapted to what we ate before cereal crops such as wheat were first cultivated around ten thousand years ago. A growing number of doctors now support that point of view too; it is no longer a fringe movement. In spite of the American Heart Association (AHA) and the American Diabetes Association (ADA) pushing the benefits of whole-grain cereals, I have certainly come to question their benefits while carrying out my investigations. Interestingly, many animals (including monkeys and apes) are not adapted to eating cereal grains either; but again … more of that later!

Let's get back to the real start of my journey. Around the turn of the twenty-first century, I had already been living for some years in California. I took the opportunity to take part in a two-week professional cookery course with the CIA – The Culinary Institute of America, that is. Chef Adam was in charge of our group of hobby and semi-professional chefs at the wonderful Greystone Mansion in St Helena. The city is situated in the magnificent Napa Valley, which is equally famous for its excellent wines and for its wonderful restaurants. As students, we found the scene somewhat similar to what you can see on MasterChef; each member of the training group had their own range of ovens, fridges, cooking and prep areas in front of them. There was a steep initial learning curve, but after that initial training our objective was to cook lunch each day for the 150 or so professional students who were attending the college. Quite a frightening prospect, at least for the first few days, but we soon got into the swing of things.

The CIA teaching techniques are based on the traditional French approach, but combine Californian and Mexican ingredients with a low-fat approach wherever possible. 'Why low-fat?' I asked. Chef Adam threw the question out to the room of twenty or so participants. I don't recall every answer, but the responses went something like this: 'Everyone knows animal fats are bad for you'; 'It's the cholesterol'; 'Eating fat makes you fat'; 'Fat has twice as many calories as protein and carbs'; 'Cooking with solid fats is gross' and so on. Chef Adam's response? That is something I do remember. With a subtle grin on his face, he said: 'Well, low-fat cooking certainly doesn't improve the taste, does it?'

Why exactly did the Americans lead us into this 'healthy' low-fat era, which started about fifty years ago? And to what degree has it worked – or not? They have certainly grown much fatter and (perhaps surprisingly) it hasn't helped them live longer. In 2015, the citizens of the United States of America dropped to place fifty-three in the global longevity rankings with an average age of 78.9 years.[2] This put them way behind Italy (where they live over three years longer) and Japan (where they enjoy a full six years of longer life). Interestingly, Americans have also not grown taller. In fact, their heights have stagnated. Over the past fifty years, they have added (on average) less than one inch while putting on about 25 pounds (12 kilos).[3] Today, they average about 5 feet 9 inches for men (1m 75cm) and 5 feet 4 inches for women (1m 63cm).[4] From the time of the American Revolution until 1950, the United States had the world's tallest individuals – but now they find themselves in place twenty-seven on the global rankings list.[5] This puts them behind countries like Spain and Belgium and way behind the Dutch, whose average male height now exceeds 6 feet (1m 83cm).[6] So, what's going on … and just how much of this is diet-related?

---

2   Geoba.se, 2015.
3   Ogden et al., 2004.
4   Idem.
5   AverageHeight.co, n.d.
6   Stulp et al., 2015.

How did we get here?

The thing is that our diets, our stomachs and the 1.5 kilos or so of bacteria living down there, aiding our digestive system, are only partly understood by researchers and specialist doctors. It turns out that further analysis of the research done in the 1960s and '70s (which led to today's low-fat, high-carb dietary recommendations) has shown that it was deeply flawed and, if anything, inconclusive. But that didn't stop the scientists and government bodies with a vested interest in issuing one or the other dietary recommendations, and it certainly didn't stop the giant food lobbies who were pushing from all sides.

The famous US *Food Guide Pyramid* went through numerous variations[7] while the lobbyists argued. Interestingly, the woman originally tasked with developing the food pyramid back in 1980, Luise Light, gave up and resigned before it finally saw the light of day in 1992. In an essay written ten years later and entitled *A Fatally Flawed Food Guide*,[8] she talked of 'a government bowing to industry interests'. She went on to suggest that those many Americans who did follow the recommended food pyramid probably ended up overweight because of it. It is certainly true that our diet and eating habits in the Western world have been greatly influenced by these guidelines, which were later emulated in the UK and many other countries. Yet the reality is that they had more to do with industry interests than healthy eating. There was (and is) no consensus on what constitutes healthy eating, and the food pyramid was pretty much based on politics rather than sound science.

Luise Light's team recommended a pyramid base with 5–9 servings of fresh fruits and vegetables a day, but this was replaced with a paltry 2–3 servings before being revised upwards to 5–7 servings a couple of years later in association with a separate anti-cancer campaign by the National Cancer Institute. Another recommendation of 3–4 daily

---

7   USDA National Agricultural Library, n.d.
8   Light, 2004.

servings of whole-grain breads and cereals was changed to 'a whopping 6–11 servings' and ended up forming the base of the *Food Guide Pyramid* instead; this was a concession to the processed wheat and corn industries.

Baked goods made with white flour (including cakes, sweets and other low-nutrient foods) had originally been put at the peak of the pyramid, with the guideline 'eat sparingly'. Yet in the 'revised' *Food Guide Pyramid* they were added to the pyramid's base. Changes were also made to the wording of the dietary guidelines from 'eat less' to 'avoid too much', which helped the processed-food industry by not limiting their fast-growing and highly profitable junk foods market segment – that could have seriously dented their bottom line. It's interesting to note how, in comparison, those 1941 guidelines illustrated in Figure 1 featured just '2 or more' servings of cereal or bread and regular egg and dairy consumption. Looking at things from where I sit today, Great-Grandma's diet seems pretty healthy.

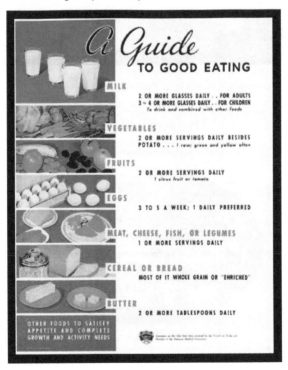

Figure 1:   1941 Poster. Should you eat like your great-grandma? Looks quite healthy, don't you think?

19

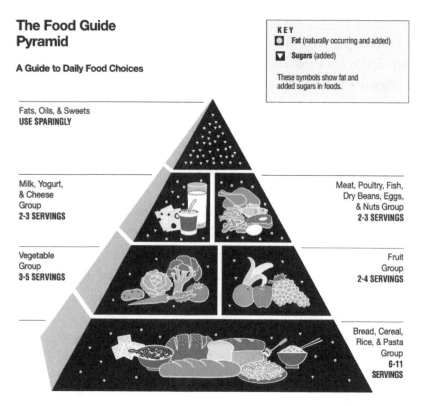

Figure 2:   The original US Food Guide Pyramid …

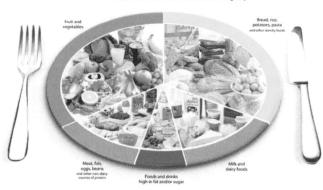

Figure 3:   … morphed into the 'eatwell plate' (NHS, UK). Fat and sugar are still lumped together in the smallest section!

Because of the proven success of 'outside interests' and lobbying groups combined with the poor quality of many nutritional studies, I view much of the standard research work as being of questionable nature and thus use very little of it in this book. (Where I *do* refer to external sources, I keep references to a minimum but provide links and also avenues for further reading in the written text.)

In taking this approach, I fully acknowledge opening myself up to the accusation of not providing scientifically grounded information. Yet the intriguing thing is this: no book or set of guidelines on diet and healthy eating is actually based on scientific principles, and no research results appear to go uncontested.

To emphasise this situation, Stanley Young, former Director of Bioinformatics at the US National Institute of Statistical Sciences, estimates that for observational studies in the medical field,[9] 'over 90% of the claims fail to replicate'. That means that they cannot be replicated later by more exacting experiments. To quote him from a talk given in 2009 to members of the Sigma Xi Science Research Society (a body of more than 80,000 scientists and engineers):[10] 'Wow. Is this really science? Every observational study could be challenged'.

That's why there is so little agreement from doctors and nutritionists on what constitutes healthy eating, and that's why so many purveyors of the next new and revolutionary diet that's 'guaranteed to help you lose pounds' can make a packet from their approach – however gimmicky – if they just get their marketing right. Most diets succeed in helping you lose weight because you eat less for a short while; it's continuing to keep the pounds off which causes the problems.

---

9   Mayo, 2013.
10   As reported by Whoriskey, 2015 (1).

Fat and your hormones

Your body doesn't like it when you try to lose a few kilos. In spite of the extra weight registered by your knees, the extra effort that your heart needs to pump blood around your body and the extra 'unhealthy' fat steadily accumulating around your internal organs, it's a different signal that wins out. When you deprive your body of the food it needs to maintain your current weight, a primitive hormonal signal is issued to try to stop you altering the current balance of fat and muscle on your body. Just when you reach for the low-fat yoghurt, hoping to enter body-fat burning mode and lose those first grams, your body says 'Just a minute!' and encourages you to maintain the status quo; to keep your 'set-point', as some nutritionists like to say.

Views differ on exactly why this is, but one of the most commonly accepted theories is that our ancestors needed to fatten up in the late summer and prepare for the scarcity of food which would occur during the winter months. Just as migrating birds stock up on food before their long flights, it is thought that we do the same before a long winter. The problem is that these days our bodies don't know when the tough times are coming, so we keep stocking up – just in case. An excess of the foods we are most likely to eat today leads to excess fat on our waists and hips. The only way of stopping that fat-making process is to trick your system. You won't do that by counting calories. That will only leave you feeling hungry and lead to a misbalance in your metabolic system – particularly if you follow the 'approved' low-fat nutritional guidelines. Ironically, one of the first things I learned was that eating fat does not make you fat. Fat is good for you in most of its different oily and solid forms, and our hormones respond positively to increased fat in the diet – as long as it's the right sort. Your hormonal balance is reaffirmed when fat replaces some of the refined flours (and particularly sugars) that we eat so much of these days in their various processed forms. Our hormones don't much like an excess of these carbohydrates – especially when, like today, it's never-ending.

When it comes to our weight, most of us are to be found in the same slimming category: we are weight-loss resistant. Yet we know that not everyone is. We all know those people who seem to eat what they want and still stay skinny. Funnily enough, from an evolutionary standpoint, they would normally be the unlucky ones. Unable in ancient hunter-gatherer societies to take advantage of those times when food was plentiful, they would not have been able to store reserves on their body in the form of fat. You could say that today they are benefiting from a hormonal defect which now protects them – but that sounds a bit cruel. If you are one of these people, this book is probably not for you – but it just might be. Many slim people are still surprisingly fat on the inside. Lathe Poland from Bethel, Connecticut, USA made a Kickstarter-funded film about this subject when he was (in his words, 'quite inexplicably') diagnosed in 2010 with type-2 diabetes. He had associated this illness with being fat on the outside. His lifestyle had him following all the doctor-endorsed guidelines, from drinking low-fat milk to regularly working out. 'I could not have been more surprised,' said the trim filmmaker, who stands just over 6 feet (1 m 83 cm) tall and weighs in at 75 kilos. 'I did not think I fit the classic model.' After trying medication for a few months he got interested in just how diabetes was affecting more and more people. The end result, if you get a chance to watch, is his entertaining and informative film, *Carb-Loaded: A Culture Dying to Eat.*[11]

Getting back to the important role of hormones: they drive both the balance and the effectiveness of your body's metabolism – it's not calories that do that. Obviously, if you want to lose weight, the amount that you eat plays a fundamental role – but it is becoming clear that the quantity is less important than the quality of what you eat. Just look at Sam Feltham's example (see insert), whereby he fattened up on processed carbohydrates (those being both starches and sugar) but did well on a high-fat diet. OK; he's a sample of one. But one of the difficulties in this world of nutrition is that there are very few examples of well-run research

11 TheSceneLab, 2014.

studies that would be readily accepted in other branches of science. As a health coach and fat loss expert, Sam Feltham now runs a successful business and you can read more about him at www.smashthefat.com.

Sam Feltham's Story

Sam Feltham runs a website called smashthefat.com. Back in February 2014, he decided to self-experiment by consuming more than 5,000 calories per day of low-carbohydrate/high-fat foods for 21 days. His diet consisted of large quantities of meat, eggs, greens and nuts, with the following average macronutrient breakdown – calories of 5,794 per day by eating: protein – 333gm; fat – 461gm; carbs – 85gm. In calorie terms, that represents a 71% fat diet.

He started by estimating his daily calorie needs at just over 3,100 – quite a high level because he cycles a lot. Using the 'calories in = calories out' approach, he should have gained about 6 kilos in those 21 days. But, he didn't. He gained just over a kilo while losing an inch (2.5cm) around his waist.

So, would the result be different if he took in over 5,000 calories daily on a diet high in refined carbohydrates (cereals, pasta, potatoes, rice, sugar etc.)? More importantly, would the hormonal effects of the carbohydrates beat out the natural resistance he had demonstrated when over-eating fat? In the next 21-day period, his diet consisted of cereals, breads, jam, pasta, desserts and sugary sodas. The daily calories added up to 5,793. By weight, this was made up of: protein – 188gm; fat – 141gm; carbs – 893gm. In calorie terms, that's a 64% carb diet.

On the final day he weighed in at 96.8kg – up 7.1 kilos on his starting weight. This was more or less what the calorie formula would have predicted with his 53,872 total calorie surplus. But, in spite of his bike riding, he did not gain muscle tissue on this carb-rich diet. He did, however, add a full 3 inches (8cm) to his waist.

Summary: when on the high-carb over-eating diet, the calorie equation held up. But, on the fat-rich diet, what Sam ate bore little relationship to his weight.

Most research results and recommendations fall into the 'correlation is not necessarily causation' category. You only have to read the *Daily Mail* to get regular updates of this kind. One week, chocolate makes you fat; the next, it's an essential nutrient. Another week goes by, and extreme vegan shakes provide the slimmer's answer. Then we're advised that butter was actually good for us and we should not have stopped eating it. Then there's the whole eggs fiasco – but don't get me started!

Although there are a few definitive linkages which result from this type of epidemiological research (statistical correlation of health in populations), such as the undisputed association between lung cancer and smoking, the weak associations between varying foods and their health consequences fall into a very different category.

We have read that these studies usually cannot be reproduced, but they are often open to easy misinterpretation – particularly by interested lobby groups. As Dr John Yudkin (nutritionist, physician and primary exponent for the idea that sugar consumption promotes heart disease) said back in the 1970s:[12] 'There is a close relationship between the number of televisions being bought and fatal heart attacks'. That didn't mean that people were being killed by their TVs. A possible interpretation might have been that their increasingly sedentary lifestyles had something to do with the data – but even that is one of many possible interpretations.

It has now become clear[13] that eating healthy dietary fat does not make you fat or ill, in spite of some earlier 'research-based' correlations which were later shown to be just that; associations that made sense to those interpreting them. However, they were taken so seriously by governments and the medical community that they are still having a significant effect on our world today.

But … we keep drifting away from the role of hormones! The essence of the 'hormones first' approach is that low-calorie diets – and particularly fat-free produce – do not help your metabolism; they disturb it and overwhelm it. Traditional dietary approaches advise you to control calories by eating an unnatural balance of chemically altered foods from

---

12   Yudkin, 1972, Chapter 13.
13   See Harcombe et al., 2015.

which fat has been removed and to which starches, sugars and emulsifiers have been added to improve taste and consistency. Even something as innocent as low-fat milk, which used to be made by removing the fat by gravity (the cream rises to the top), is now made by placing the natural milk in a machine called a centrifugal separator, which spins some or all of the fat globules out of the milk. Then the milk is homogenised; a process which reduces all the milk particles to the same size so that natural separation no longer occurs. Next (at least in the USA), it is fortified with vitamins A and D, since those vitamins are fat-soluble and they were lost during the skimming process. Milk solids in the form of dried milk solids are then added to thicken the watery consistency of the skimmed milk. In spite of this, semi-skimmed milk (about 2% fat) is the most-sold milk in the USA. Similar semi-skimmed milk (about 1.5% fat; vs whole milk which is about 3.5% fat) is the most popular milk sold in the UK. My niece tells me off when I don't have 'normal' milk in the fridge. You can't imagine how much that upsets me! She and many others are convinced that whole milk is not 'full-fat' but 'full-of-fat', and that drinking it will lead to fatty arteries and an early death. Putting it politely: what a load of codswallop. Yet, having said that, it's not her fault. Years of government health guidelines, well-meaning dieticians and 'big-food' advertisements have combined to brainwash her into thinking that whole milk is unhealthy – yet the research is simply not there to back up that supposition. Quite the opposite, in fact, considering that the body's vitamin and calcium absorption rates diminish when less fat is present. My views, too, have changed. When I started working on this investigative project, I would also order my low-fat cappuccinos – thinking that this would reduce my intake of fat, cholesterol and calories. Now I know that I was wrong; such a simplistic approach is incorrect.

The problem is that using artificially altered foods (even healthy sounding, low-fat milk) confuses your metabolism. At their worst, diets featuring an array of today's chemically changed products lead to weight gain and disease – notably type-2 diabetes – and contribute to numerous auto-immune disorders and allergies. Most low-fat yoghurts contain a concoction of chemical emulsifiers to thicken them combined with artificial sweeteners (or corn-based sugars) to add back some taste. Some of these ingredients are untested on humans and many are used in industrial products and animal food. These highly processed products fail to even switch on the hormonal systems which register that you are getting full; put briefly, they short-circuit the appetite-suppressing effects of the hormone leptin.

According to Daniel Goleman, who writes on the subject of emotional intelligence:[14] 'Whenever we feel stressed out, that's a signal that our brain is pumping out stress hormones. If sustained over months and years, those hormones can ruin our health and make us a nervous wreck'. But your hormones also determine how you feel when it comes to hunger and cravings. This creates a different kind of stress. Insulin (controlling blood glucose levels), leptin (suppressing appetite) and ghrelin (increasing appetite) are the three main hormones that influence hunger. Ghrelin also has an impact on when you feel cravings for one particular food or another. Cortisol, dopamine and serotonin – which affect your mood and general 'feel-good' factor – also play a role, but it's the way all these hormones interplay which provides your body with feedback (in the form of stress or pangs of hunger, for example). Yet this feedback system is currently being undermined by the strange cocktail of processed foods that most of us eat these days. Compare, as Dr John Emsley does,[15] the list of seventeen ingredients on the packet of supposedly healthy Flora Light margarine with the one ingredient (namely, cream) which goes into supposedly unhealthy butter. Is it any wonder that your digestive system, fine-tuned by thousands of years of evolution, gets a bit confused?

A further example of this confusion can be found in your levels of the hormone leptin (which you'll remember suppresses your appetite). This should normally be lower when you're thinner and higher when you've put on some weight. However, a growing number of people seem to have built up resistance to the appetite-suppressing effects of leptin. It's all to

---

14   Goleman, 1995, Chapter 2: *Anatomy of an Emotional Hijacking.*
15   Emsley, 2012.

do with the complicated interaction between your gut and your brain. As yet, nobody – not even the world's top researchers – understands it fully.

When functioning correctly, leptin (which is secreted by your fat cells) sends a signal to your brain saying that there is currently sufficient stored energy. In other words, you don't need to eat. What seems to happen with time is that people with a lot of body fat (who regularly, over months and years, secrete high levels of leptin into their bloodstream) somehow confuse their brain into no longer registering the leptin. The 'blinded' brain believes that they are still hungry. This resistance to leptin has been found to be one of the leading reasons that obese people struggle to lose weight. If you are one of the increasing number of leptin-resistant people out there, what's happening is that the other hormones are joining forces to successfully drive your increased food intake. It's a bit like being in a car with a failing brake pedal. Trying to exert your willpower against that malfunctioning, leptin-driven starvation signal is very difficult. This allows insulin to take over the driver's seat. Insulin is, after all, the major energy storage hormone in the body. What it does is signal to your cells that they need to store energy (in the form of either glycogen or fat) even when they don't need it. Glycogen builds up and is stored in the liver, but there is only a limited capacity. Such constant overwork can lead to fatty liver disease – a fast-growing ailment today even among the younger members of society. Because of this, the American Nutrition Science Initiative (NuSI) is currently running a randomised, controlled clinical trial to help determine whether removing added sugars from the diets of children can stop or reverse such non-alcoholic fatty liver disease.[16] Putting glycogen to one side, our body's capacity to store energy in the form of fat, when not hormonally reined in, is (as we all know) immense. That's why so many of us are putting on the pounds.

So, cut some slack to any overweight person you know who goes on a semi-starvation diet (or a series of them) – which is what calorie-reduction programmes effectively are. The mental and physical struggle that they are going through is much greater than if you are of regular

16   NuSI, n.d.

weight and are just choosing to lose a couple of pounds. We can see it, but they genuinely feel it.

Mr and Mrs Overweight who visit their doctor will still generally be told to 'cut back on the calories'. This forces them into the low-fat trap. They'll be asked to eat a healthy, balanced diet. Reference will be made to whole grains, but there will not be a word spoken about avoiding processed foods. Is this because it's considered too difficult for most of us to do? No-one seems to agree on the best definition of a balanced diet, in any case, but I think that Grant Schofield, who's Professor of Public Health in Auckland, New Zealand gets close with:[17] 'A balanced diet is one which normalises blood glucose and prevents the hyper-secretion of insulin'.

That's exactly what a low-carbohydrate, high-fat diet does for you. It helps you regain control of the hormonal balance which regulates your body's fat storage capabilities. If you follow the guidelines in this book, I believe that you can gain a healthier body and mind, experience better digestive processes and have a happier disposition – which all sounds a bit too good to be true, doesn't it? But it gets better. Over time, you will also steadily reduce weight. However, there is (yes, I repeat) no one-size-fits-all solution. Each one of us is different. Although the principles remain the same, you will need to modify the precise details of your diet to get things just right for you – but that is not complex or difficult. Put simply: **to have a positive hormonal effect on your body, you will need to stop dieting** (at least in the sense that most of us understand that word today) and **begin your new life by eating naturally**. If you combine that new eating approach with some light exercise, such as taking a brisk walk, your whole body will benefit. And if you choose to go further with exercise, that's fine – but it is not the major contributor when it comes to steady and sustainable weight loss. My sister-in-law, Katy, lost 20 kilos with this dietary approach. But, more importantly, she now takes pleasure in walking up the two flights of stairs at work – something that used to be a real effort. That's the sort of real-life exercise

---

17   Schofield, 2015.

situation that makes a difference; each body is its own finely tuned ecosystem, and everyone's experience will be slightly different.

A word on inflammation

You'll find the word 'inflammation' referred to several times in this book, both in the context of what you eat and in terms of what that food does to your body. After the apparently misguided focus of the last fifty years or so on the evils of consuming fat and the dangers of having high cholesterol levels, medical opinion is slowly coming round to the idea that inflammation is at the root of a lot of chronic disease today. Too much stress is one of the many factors that cause inflammation, which in turn can all too easily affect your heart – or so the hypothesis goes. That's the official viewpoint of the American Heart Association. An extract from their website reads:[18] 'Although it is not proven that inflammation causes cardiovascular disease, inflammation is common for heart disease and stroke patients and is thought to be a sign of atherogenic (the process of forming plaques in the inner lining of arteries) response'.

So, in this context, what exactly does inflammation refer to? When, for example, you bump yourself hard against a counter top, it results in a dark-coloured bruise. That swelling or inflammation represents your body's natural defence mechanism coming to the rescue. In that particular case, the swollen area around a bruise or a cut draws blood to the area and contributes to a faster healing process – so it's a good thing! But when too much inflammation takes place within your body, it is being increasingly linked to poor health outcomes; most typically to cardiovascular disease (meaning heart attacks and strokes). Unlike a bruise, you do not notice it until the increased cellular damage has accumulated and led to one of today's chronic diseases such as obesity, diabetes, heart disease, cancer or Alzheimer's – but an increasing number of doctors are attributing the ultimate cause of these diseases to cellular inflammation. Those proponents argue that cellular inflammation initiates chronic disease because it disrupts the body's natural hormonal signalling networks.

---

18   American Heart Association, 2015.

Today's researchers are spending more time on the subject. A recent study shows how they are now gaining increased knowledge about the processes involved. One of the lead investigators, Daniel Capelluto, an associate professor and research fellow in the Virginia Bioinformatics Institute, commented:[19] 'The inflammatory response can be a double-edged sword. At appropriate levels, the inflammatory response protects your body from foreign materials, but if it is not properly regulated it can lead to severe, chronic conditions'.

Admittedly, reducing mental stress is one factor that leads to less inflammation in the body and that will potentially help lead you to a longer life. However, there are also many other contributors to be found in the textbooks. Doctors speak of poor air quality and general high levels of pollution. Most frequently, however, they bring up (not literally!) the food you eat every single day of your life. In terms of impact on your body, nothing is likely to beat food; its effects accumulate steadily over your entire lifespan. To get an idea of just how much you eat in your lifetime, try picturing a male African elephant (the largest land mammal). It stands at nearly four metres in height and weighs in at over 5 to 6,000 kilos. In your lifetime, you will eat the equivalent weight of at least six such elephants. Put in that light, it should be no surprise to discover that the food we eat every day contributes significantly to our wellbeing and particularly to the degree of inflammation accumulating in our bodies.

When it comes to visiting the doctor, most of us deal with time-starved general practitioners who treat our medical concerns one at a time and don't look at the big picture. Qualified holistic medical doctors are something of a luxury, but if you can find one (and if you can afford them) they represent money well spent. They carry out a form of treatment that considers the whole person – including your body, mind, spirit, emotions, diet and living environment – all in the search for optimal health. They try to help you achieve a proper balance in your life. Doctors such as Cate Shanahan, author of *Deep Nutrition*[20] (now

---

19   Virginia Tech, 2015.
20   Shanahan, 2009.

based in Denver, Colorado), and consultant to the LA Lakers basketball team include an anti-inflammatory lifestyle diet 'particularly designed to prevent inflammation in your internal organs' as an important part of their treatment programme.[21] Funnily enough, your grandma also knew something about inflammation when she advised you to take a tablespoon of cod liver oil (which is rich in omega-3 fatty acids) before you left the house. OK, she may not have known why – but she was actually at the cutting edge of dietary advice on the subject of inflammation. We all know that today's typical fast food meal contains large quantities of refined, starchy carbohydrates in the form of burger buns and fries, but there is also a high level of omega-6 fatty acids to be found – mostly as a result of the ubiquitous vegetable seed oils that we use so much of today. This is not really surprising when you consider that when mixed together these ingredients make up the cheapest source of calories known to mankind – and they can also make foods such as fried chicken and French fries taste great. Today's industrialised beef, chicken and pork products are also much richer in omega-6 fatty acids. This is largely as a result of the animal fattening process and the feedstuffs used. The problem for your body (and, in particular, your digestive tract) is that they are all highly inflammatory. Nothing has an effect on the inflammation inside your body – the invisible kind – more than the type of oil you eat. Fish oils, many nuts and free range animal meats contain a higher proportion of omega-3 fatty acids whereas seed oils (often wrongly named as vegetable oils and made, for example, from corn, soy and sunflower) contain none. Omega-6 fatty acids make up more than half of the content of such seed oils. Yet, in evolutionary terms, there has never been a time when we have eaten substantially more omega-6 than omega-3 oils.

Taking a historical perspective, we currently appear to be way out of balance. This is simply because all these extracted seed oils did not even exist before the start of the twentieth century. Back then, animal fats such as lard, beef tallow and (of course) butter were what we used in the kitchen. If you increase the amount of omega-3 that you consume, less

---

21   See www.drcate.com

omega-6 will be available to your bodily tissues to produce inflammation. While omega-6 is pro-inflammatory, omega-3 is neutral. That is why a diet featuring a high proportion of omega-6 and containing only small quantities of omega-3 will increase inflammation. Interestingly, the way over-the-counter pain-killers such as ibuprofen and aspirin work is by reducing the formation of inflammatory compounds derived from omega-6 fatty acids. Why not consider simply limiting your dietary intake of omega-6 rich oils to help cure your pain? It's cheaper and healthier, but it is certainly not what most of today's dieticians and nutrition experts recommend. Although they generally advocate fish oil (often as a supplement in the form of daily pills), they still recommend corn and sunflower as the best cooking oils. Remember: each time you eat a potato chip/crisp, about 30% of the calories you take in are from the oil they are fried in. In the UK, that's sunflower oil. In the USA, it's more likely to be corn or soy seed oil.

Weighing and measuring

Time to get practical. When it comes to weight, your measuring stick will not be the bathroom scales. Use them for information if you wish, but when your goal is to lose some of the fat on your body, the regular measurement of your waist and hips will provide you with a much better scale. Dropping a couple of dress sizes or not being embarrassed by the waist size listed on the outside label of your Levi's 501s are the really important measures! The simple fact is that if you lose weight and your waist measurement decreases, you are losing mostly fat – congratulations! But just the same can be true if your weight goes up a bit while your waistline slims; this might be what happens to you. We are all different and our bodies sometimes go about things in slightly different ways; each of us offers up a unique and finely tuned ecosystem to the world. By the way, according to the useful guide on the Australian Heart Foundation website,[22] to consistently measure your waist in the same place, you should locate the top of your hip bone and the bottom of your ribs. Then, place your tape measure midway between these points and just wrap it around your waist. Now you know!

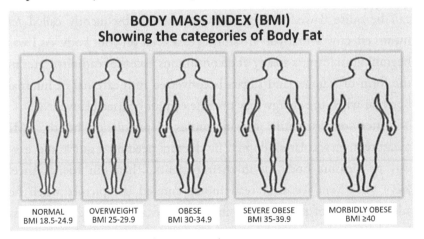

BODY MASS INDEX (BMI)
Showing the categories of Body Fat

| NORMAL BMI 18.5-24.9 | OVERWEIGHT BMI 25-29.9 | OBESE BMI 30-34.9 | SEVERE OBESE BMI 35-39.9 | MORBIDLY OBESE BMI ≥40 |

Figure 4:   Is obese becoming the new normal?

---

22   Australian Heart Foundation, n.d.

Using everyone's current favourite measure of body fat percentage, namely the BMI (Body Mass Index), is a poor indicator for many of us – simply because it was never designed to determine body fat in the first place. Derived from a simple mathematical formula, the BMI system was devised by a Belgian, Adolphe Quetelet, in the 1830s – now there's another name to add to your list of famous Belgians!

Born in what is now the Flemish part of the country, he got his doctorate in mathematics from the University of Ghent at the young age of twenty-three before founding the astronomical observatory in Brussels, which is still used to this day. His greatest interest, though, was in people and their physiques. To this end, he came up with the BMI measurement in 1832 as a way of measuring and segmenting groups of people in his statistical analyses. Having noted that weight tends to increase in relation to people's height in metres squared, he developed a simple measure for classifying people's weight/height ratio relative to an ideal weight for their height. But ... never once did he use this to provide information about body fat percentages. This was first done by American life insurance companies in the 1950s after the acceptance that overweight and mortality figures were correlated. The BMI scale is supposed to estimate how *fat* you are by dividing your weight in kilograms by your height in metres squared – but that measurement can be quite flawed. Being overweight and subsequently called *fat* means effectively that you are storing excess fat on your body. As I was beginning to learn, a steady and continuous excess of carbohydrates in the form of starches and sugars is converted into external or internal body fat when the energy they provide cannot be used elsewhere.

After some scientific use in studies of population health, BMI measurement was later adopted by doctors needing a quick and easy way to measure body fat in their patients. Then our friend Ancel Keys (of whom we shall read more) entered the picture when he advocated use of the Quetelet index. He renamed it the Body Mass Index in the process and called it the best of the available indices of obesity.[23] By 1985, the American National Institute of Health began

23   Keys et al., 1972.

defining obesity according to BMI, and the overweight thresholds were established at 27.8 for men and 27.3 for women. In 1998, these figures were consolidated for men and women even though their BMI/body fat relationship is quite different. In addition, thresholds were lowered; they were now defined as being 25 for overweight and 30 for obesity. In the USA, where this redefinition took place, the immediate effect was the re-allocation of approximately twenty-nine million Americans from the 'healthy' category to the 'overweight' category. A conspiracy theorist might add that many of those on the 'independent' board making the recommendations for these new lower cut-off levels had connections to the commercial weight-loss industry and stood to profit financially, but …

Nevertheless, the simple fact is that two people with the same BMI can have quite different weights and distributions of body fat so that a direct correlation with heart disease and type-2 diabetes is still only indicative. BMI measurements also have no way of distinguishing between fat and muscle content. This means that, for example, many ultra-fit international level rugby players would qualify as being obese. Admittedly, today, with so many people around the world reaching the 'severely obese' or 'morbidly obese' categories, this point is becoming rather academic.

As a result of all this, my experience has shown that waist and hip measurements are better and more reliable indicators of dietary progress; weight fluctuates on a daily basis and should be measured weekly. Let's put things bluntly: your body's normal full digestive process (from eating to pooping) takes thirty to forty hours, and your body's water retention can vary by more than a kilo per day; so don't weigh yourself daily – it's pretty meaningless.

Government guidelines and 'nutritionism'

The government- and health service-endorsed guidelines relating to what we eat and how much we exercise tend to put us all in the same boat, and ask us to shift our sails in the same modified dietary direction if we want to achieve weight loss. A solid dietary starting point, however, necessitates that these guidelines must be scientifically justified to provide us with a benchmark for our dietary journey. However, we all know that different approaches work for different people. Just as Bach introduced melodic variations into his fugues, or a modern-day jazz trumpeter will improvise around a basic theme, our individual bodies and lifestyles call for variation. And when it comes to food and drink, such variations can also provoke a different set of outcomes.

That degree of variation would be all well and good as long as those government-sponsored basic guidelines provided us with a useful starting point and were based on solid nutritional research. But, sadly enough, they are not. The current 'low-fat eating' guidelines were developed with more of an eye on their political and economic impact than on what has been demonstrated to be scientifically successful. In fact, with all the difficulties involved in putting together credible research in the field of nutrition, it may well be that there is no hard and fast way to prove the efficacy of one approach to eating over another. Very few 'in-depth' trials last for more than a few months, and the longer term effects are often simply extrapolated to try and prove a point. However, in the USA there are a couple of research projects which have become cross-generational, and these continue to provide useful data when it comes to those long-term effects of certain dietary preferences and habits. The Framingham Heart Study[24] is one of them. Based in the small town of Framingham, in Massachusetts, the study began in 1948 with 5,209 adult subjects. It is now on its third generation of participants. The latest research output[25]

---

24   Framingham Heart Study, n.d. (1).
25   Petroni, 2015.

considers that drinking sweetened soft drinks (such as cola) over many years increases the chance of fatty liver disease. Controlling people's diets over the long term and being sure of their strict adherence to the controls is difficult; some would say nigh on impossible. Furthermore, the short-term effects of various diets are usually not significant when you examine the same group of participants a year later. Because of all this, developing reliable research-based policy is not easy.

Governments use incentives of many different kinds to support their food policies. What we saw in the post-WW2 era is that subsidies were used to build up supplies of corn and wheat – the aim being to reduce the impact of any potential drought.[26] With that background, it is no wonder that the initial food pyramid had such a focus on bread, cereal, rice and pasta! The trouble is that in the USA (and elsewhere) many of these subsidies are still in place today. What we believe about healthy eating is, at least to some extent, influenced by the huge lobbying funds that get spent each year. In the UK, many of those in their forties or fifties will have noticed that more and more fields of bright yellow rapeseed have appeared over the years. European Union subsidies changed back in the 1980s to support a switch to rapeseed for a number of political reasons – including incentivising French farmers to remove poor quality vineyards and encouraging rapeseed for use as biodiesel. Some creative rapeseed entrepreneurs may be trying to encourage you to get a taste for their refined salad oils – but thanks to the EU subsidies, rapeseed currently makes up 80% of all the vegetable oil used in European biofuels.[27]

That post-WW2 environment (combined with misinterpretations of the research data on subjects like fat intake and cholesterol levels) has led, albeit indirectly, to a vast processed food industry that's based on starches (notably wheat and maize), sugars and huge quantities of seed oils made from the likes of corn, soy and sunflowers. We, the customers, have gained the convenience factor of snacking 'on the go', eating out cheaply and being able to pop pre-prepared dishes in the microwave. But

---

26   See Fields, 2004.
27   See Gilbert, 2012.

we have sacrificed, at least to some degree, our health. What is becoming clearer every day is that our sacrifice is bigger than we ever imagined.

'Compounding the problem is that fattening foods are supported whereas healthy fare isn't,' says Barry Popkin, Professor of Nutrition at the University of North Carolina.[28] 'We put maybe one-tenth of one percent of our dollar that we put into subsidizing and promoting foods through the Department of Agriculture into fruits and vegetables. As a result, the price gap between high-sugar, high-fat foods and more nutritionally valuable fruits and vegetables is artificially large. That means in supermarkets and restaurants, red meats, sugar-and fat-loaded products, and fast foods not only appear to be the best buys but in proportion to even moderate salaries are downright cheap.'

Just for the record, the subsidized 'high-sugar, high-fat' foods that Professor Popkin refers to contain high-fructose corn syrup (made from maize) and vegetable seed oils (largely extracted from soy, corn and peanuts). The 'cheap' red meat represents cattle fed with a surplus of cheap grain. The situation is not so extreme in Europe, but the principles are the same. According to the Organization for Economic Cooperation and Development (OECD) figures,[29] the average rate of 'producer support estimate' for the heavily supported commodities in the United States ranges from about 55% of the value of production for sugar to about 22% percent for oilseeds. For the less-supported commodities, the rate is typically below 5%.[30]

Conventional medical wisdom, particularly in the USA, likes to refer to something called the 'French paradox'. The thinking behind this is along these lines: how can those Southern Europeans eat such fatty diets and drink red wine and still live longer and healthier lives than we do on our 'healthy' diets over here? Perhaps a better question is: why, after years of advice, have our 'Western' diets not led to us becoming healthier citizens? Let's take a closer look at our daily food intake. The nutritionists have given their stamp of approval to a wide

---

28   Cited by Fields, 2004, Chapter: *From Farm Fields to Grocery Bills*.
29   OECD, 2007, p.49.
30   Sumner, 2008.

range of processed convenience foods by using a reductionist chemistry-set based approach to health. Sugar Pops not good for you? Just add some vitamins! Low-fat milk not quite doing the trick? Just add some different vitamins! Greek yoghurt too high in fat, but people love the taste and the thicker texture? Just add some chemical emulsifiers and a bit of sugar! Pork too high in omega-6 fat? Start feeding them on omega-3 rich foods! If only it were all as simple as that.

'Nutritionism' is the word given to this reduction and measurement of foods into their component parts. But to think that synthetic vitamins are just the same as naturally occurring ones is simplistic and incorrect; to think that an individual 'rice crispie' is the nutritional equivalent of a grain of rice? Whether you eat flakes of corn or crisps of rice, a number of health benefits are usually claimed for such breakfast cereals depending on their fortification with 'essential minerals' and synthetic vitamins. Even the added sugar is usually portrayed as giving you energy. Yet the original micronutrients from the raw ingredients were either destroyed by the process or stripped away before it – leaving (funnily enough) the calorific value just the same. In his 1982 book, *Fighting the Food Giants*,[31] biochemist Paul Stitt describes the cereal grain extrusion process, which treats the grains with very high heat and pressure. He goes on to explain how the processing denatures the fatty acids, damages the amino acid lysine and even destroys the synthetic vitamins added at the end of the process. The amino acid lysine, a crucial nutrient, is especially damaged by the extrusion process. So, to say that a single corn flake which has endured much heat and physical turbulence is nutritionally just the same as a fresh kernel of corn has proven to be naïve at best. Yet the way such nutritional information is listed on the label of the box will still make you feel quite good about what you are eating – as long as you quickly skip those sugar percentages! For much more information on this topic, if you don't find it too depressing, I suggest reading *Eat Your Heart Out*.[32] This is an informative book by Felicity Lawrence, published in 2008.

---

31   Stitt, 1982.
32   Lawrence, 2008.

Current food labelling provides us with many examples of this reductionism, with a can of cola equalling a kilo of celery (when you count the calories) or an apple being seen as the equivalent of two teaspoons of sugar. Not surprisingly, when it comes to advertising and marketing, companies such as Coca-Cola admit to working with a network of dieticians and bloggers to reinforce their message. Coca-Cola says that it wants to:[33] 'help people make decisions that are right for them', and that – like others in the industry – it works with health experts 'to help bring context to the latest facts and science around [its] products and ingredients'. But ... which lobbyists are speaking up for the bunch of celery? Who is advocating the less profitable fresh ingredients? I see no nutritional content stickers on fresh vegetables, fruit, meat or eggs and only the occasional mention of anti-inflammatory omega-3 fatty acids when it comes to fresh fish.

Focusing on calories and on macro- and micro-nutrients risks not seeing the wood for the trees. The truth is not only that the subject of what we eat is much more complex than we thought; in addition, we are only just beginning to understand the power of many of the digestive interactions that follow. Ben Goldacre, the British doctor and science writer, has declared in the *New Statesman* that:[34] 'nutritionism' is the 'bollocks du jour' and that it is 'driven by a set of first year undergraduate errors in interpreting scientific data'. I must admit that I now go some way towards sharing his opinion that 'the primary promoters of nutritionism are health food manufacturers, self-proclaimed gurus and journalists who have an incomplete understanding of science, along with a credulous public that is willing to believe whatever simplistic theories they are told in the mass media'.

Being aware that you might by now think that I'm in the process of setting myself up as a 'self-proclaimed guru', let me set 'nutritionism' to one side and consider whether the much-touted French paradox (or Mediterranean paradox, for that matter), which shows the French, Spanish and Italians living longer, healthier lives free of heart disease in

33   Choi, 2015.
34   Goldacre, 2007.

spite of their diet, is the real norm. What if those Southern Europeans are healthier … *because* of their 'rich' diet? These questions, when I first became interested in them, soon led me to Southern Italy and the small hillside town of Roseto – but more of that later.

What if the true paradox is to question why, in the USA, the UK and (to a slightly lesser extent) central Europe, we have developed a diet that consists of pre-prepared, packaged and processed junk food of low nutritional value. We just love to eat our boxed cereals, ready-made meals, chicken nuggets, fries and hamburgers served in fluffy carb-loaded buns made from flour which has had all its goodness removed. Why, even in the poorest parts of Southern Italy, do women today live four years longer on average than women in the USA? The question is: where is the real paradox? Just because some poorly interpreted research data from the middle of the twentieth century led crusading scientists to demonise traditional cooking methods and fats such as butter and lard, we have ended up with a food industry that has us putting on the pounds and increasingly suffering from chronic illnesses such as type-2 diabetes. The only ones to benefit are the drug companies that square the circle with their prescription supplies of pills and insulin, those managing the many weight-loss programmes on offer and – more recently, perhaps – the expanding fitness tracker business.

There are so many differing diet and exercise plans on the market, all designed to help us lose weight. 'Before' and 'after' photos are often used to support claims about calorie-controlled diets, but if you are to be genuinely successful in the long term, you need to consider the continuing, maintenance stage. When America and its allies invaded Iraq and ousted Saddam Hussein in 2003, they may have won the war, but they did not consider either the immediate repercussions or the longer term future. OK; that may be an an analogy too far, but why start a diet without considering the future? Why eat one special way only to return to your previous ways of eating some weeks or months later? It should not be about short-term weight loss, but keeping the pounds and kilos off for ever – and yet reports show that less than 5% of diets bring long-term success. Although – as mentioned already several times

– while there is no one-size-fits-all diet that will work for everyone, there are certain basic guidelines which do allow us to eat well, lose weight and then maintain that new weight and body shape.

Weight, genetics and a harmful food culture

Many of us want to lose a bit of weight, but whether it's a question of a few pounds or a more dramatic shift that involves dropping several sizes in clothing, you will know by now that learning to eat well is a critical part of the recipe for success ... *before* you start to diet. Often the two will work hand in hand, but by taking that first step, you are beginning the process of investing in a longer, healthier life. Investing in the future you – but also (importantly) the current, present YOU. According to Benjamin Franklin, the only things certain in life are death and taxes. So, putting taxes to one side, let's picture a visionary, long-term goal for life and describe it as 'dying young, but as late as you can'. Imagine leading a long life, free from chronic illnesses, aches and pains. Imagine staying mobile and independent, in full control of your faculties, until you have reached a ripe old age. And what if a relatively simple set of dietary changes was likely to be the secret to this longer, healthier life? Today, many people in their twenties and thirties already experience a lack of energy or suffer from relatively harmless but debilitating illnesses such as IBS and inexplicable skin conditions. Lactose and gluten intolerances are on the rise, as are many other unidentifiable allergies. Pills are being prescribed like never before – many of them helping to balance blood sugar levels for type-2 diabetes or working in other ways to counter the effects of our Western diet.

But ... how healthy we are is all down to genetics and luck, I hear you say? Not according to Professor Tim Spector, Professor of Genetics at London's King's College University. His considered view[35] is that your environment and all it encompasses – from where you live to what you eat, or from the influence of your friends to how many times you were prescribed with antibiotics as a child – almost always has more influence on your health than the genes with which you were born. Yes, nature predetermines a lot, but nurture determines more – including the ability

---

35 Spector, 2012, Chapter: *Introduction.*

to switch on and off some of those inherited genes in your body. In particular, the study of twins shows us that in the 'nature vs nurture' debate, both have their role to play in shaping who we become. Tim Spector has a database of over fifty thousand such twins. Psychological traits and personality are one part of the nature/nurture spectrum, but it's the food we eat that has such a major impact on our health and, of course, on the shape of our bodies – and our weight. During our lifespan, as mentioned earlier, we eat something like the equivalent of six adult male African elephants (over 30 tons of food), so the huge influence that our daily food has should not surprise us. That being said, evidence shows that we don't all respond in precisely the same way to the same foods. Genes play an important role in deciding how tolerant or intolerant we are to the lactic acid found in dairy produce, and control how much amylase our bodies produce to help us digest bread – but they provide only part of the answer to the dietary conundrums that surround us.

Don't be disturbed that factors outside your control, such as your genetic makeup, play an important role in making you who you are. After all, there is nothing in science telling you that you do not have the opportunity to exercise free will. None of us are slaves to our genes and we have varying capacities for self-control which can be strengthened or weakened by social and internal factors. Yet exercising self-control is often easier said than done. Ever run to the cookie jar because you're feeling sad? Or maybe the wine bottle? And as we have read, if our hormones are out of balance, subjects like craving and hunger become even more difficult to deal with.

When it comes down to it, there is a big difference between someone telling you what to do (which we instinctively don't like) and deciding to embark on a positive course of action yourself. This book lays out a plan for how you can take greater control over your body both in the inner terminology of mental strength and in its physical appearance. Your genes may be something you are born with (obviously), but they don't rule your life. As Tim Spector writes, they merely exert an influence. In the end, your ability to take control is greater than you may think. Put simply: you don't need to be a slave to your genes – or to anyone else's views, for that matter.

So, in this book, what I will *not* tell you is what to do. But I will recommend that it's time to take charge of your body – if you are not already doing so today – and not be a slave to what the food industry and the diet dictocrats have to say. Whatever the likes of Nestlé, Coca-Cola or Kellogg's might proclaim, their one overriding goal is to generate a return on investment for their investors. I am not suggesting for one minute that they intentionally want to make anyone sick, but you will not find 'making a healthy contribution to your individual wellbeing and to society' listed anywhere in their corporate mission statement. There is nothing wrong with that, as far as I'm concerned, as long as there are checks and balances in place in the form of the necessary guidelines and regulations to support society's aspirational goal of steadily improving life in all ways possible. But it appears that all too often, this is where things break down; at least when it comes to food governance and healthy eating doctrine.

A certain 'concours de circonstances' (roughly translated as 'shit happens', or more politely as 'the decisions which lead to unforeseen consequences') occurred in post-war USA. It has led us steadily down a pathway towards a society where processed and junk food have taken over as the principal components of our diet – at least in many parts of the Western world. The food culture in which we live today is doing us harm. Ironically, to counterbalance the harm, a huge pharmaceutical industry has grown up – ostensibly to right the wrongs of the junk food industry. The worst legacy of this strange, symbiotic partnership is to be found in the US, closely followed by the UK and those island dependencies of both that have relatively quickly moved from local produce to a Western diet within a generation. Pacific islands make up nine of the ten most obese countries in the world (according to *The Times of India*[36]), not surprisingly accompanied by some of the highest rates of type-2 diabetes, cancer and heart disease. In these islands, the traditional ways of eating were set aside in the second half of the twentieth century

36   IANS, 2015.

as their populations fully embraced an American lifestyle. Completing this Top Ten in 2014, incidentally, is Kuwait, where a fast-food culture has also become the norm in recent years. The consequence? Stomach stapling procedures are now increasingly popular in Kuwait, with enough demand to prompt, in 2014, the country's first conference for medical professionals involved in weight loss surgery. Apparently, the number of bariatric surgeons in Kuwait has increased tenfold over the past decade, with at least five thousand patients receiving the procedure – compared, for example, with just three thousand in Canada, which has thirty times the population.

But let's take a step back. The stomach stapling industry, whereby people willingly have their capacity to eat food reduced, is just the latest example of that symbiotic relationship that exists between big pharma, hospitals and the food industries. You eat too much? We'll give you the drugs to combat diabetes. You're still eating too much? Well, we can provide the facilities to operate on your stomach, and you'll lose weight simply because now you cannot physically eat as much as you'd like to. Then, we will provide surgery to reduce the amounts of flapping skin generated by the rapid weight loss … and then?

PART 2
KATY'S STORY

Getting started

As you may remember, my sister-in-law Katy was obese. At 1m 60cm and weighing in at around 100 kilos, she had given up on willpower, drugs and diets and made her first approaches to the bariatric surgeons. Her exasperated GP supported this approach. 'Nothing else works' he said after a series of failed diet attempts of the calorie-counting variety. There were three types of procedure to be considered, ranging from adjustable gastric bands through shortened intestines to complete gastric bypasses, which Katy told me were referred to as the 'gold standard'. Prices for such operations can be as cheap as $3,000 in Mexico and Venezuela, I am reliably informed, but she was looking at a state-sponsored deal in Belgium, where she lives. That still would have set her back many thousands of Euros, simply because the best surgeons will only work in certain hospitals that charge more for private rooms; thus providing a further intertwining of relationships between disease, health and money-making.

I was dead-set against it. 'He's just a cheapskate,' I can hear you thinking. But no … it wasn't about the money. It was because my sister-in-law Katy loved food. Together, we had enjoyed many non-gluttonous dining experiences with my wife and our extended family and friends. After such an operation, you are left with a small stomach sack which needs feeding with regular small doses of food. Restaurant dining in the European sense flies out of the window, and for months after the operation, you are put on a diet of liquids and purees supplemented by various vitamins. The positive side, of course, is that rapid weight loss provides a definitive, 100% guaranteed end-result – but slightly less encouraging was the news that additional operations might be necessary to remove surplus skin. That being said, Katy's doctor was adamant that – considering her high blood sugar levels (even though she was now taking Metformin, the most widely prescribed first medicine for type-2 diabetes) and her poor success rate with previous dietary attempts – she had now run out of options. The risks associated with diabetes (such as blindness, possible amputations and a higher risk of Alzheimer's) were certainly not to be laughed at. So, on balance, Katy was poised to go ahead. And this is where I decided to make my move.

I had long been interested in food and nutrition but more from the cooking side than the academic study of foodstuffs and digestion. My short course at the CIA (The Culinary Institute of America) in the Napa Valley had opened my eyes to restaurant techniques and certain professional skills, but I remained an amateur. My interest in Katy's case was piqued because of a growing sense of awareness that something strange was going on with our whole approach to food and nourishment. At the age of sixty, I am old enough to look back at how food was prepared for me by my parents and grandparents, as well as seeing how my own children, nieces and nephews deal with cooking food for themselves and their young families. I have also found myself in recent years surrounded by a growing number of people with food intolerances, sensitivities, allergies and in some cases just plain pickiness when it comes to eating. Combine this with the general exposure to a fattening society, and Katy's case simply tipped the balance for me. I had to find out more. I had to help – or at least try.

It was in May of 2012 that I made the decision to dedicate the next few months to the study of nutrition and diets. My first aim was to see if I could work with Katy to seek out an alternative dietary solution. Unsurprisingly, the Internet was my first port of call and, seeing that it was the possible consequences of type-2 diabetes that worried her the most, I began by trawling the diabetes forums. The richest source of information came from bloggers and other correspondents in the USA, and it was here that I first became aware of the large differences between the official viewpoints and the users'/sufferers' stories. Supported by the views of a small but growing fringe group of doctors, the successful weight-loss success stories that also resulted in a normalisation of blood sugar levels were directly linked to low-carbohydrate dietary approaches. That would mean cutting out starches and sugars. This was most surprising because my very first investigations had begun with the website of Diabetes

UK. Their main dietary feature at the time was 'everything you need to know about healthy baking'. Something wasn't adding up. Yet, even as I finalise this book (three years later), their recipe of the month is a Pear and Almond Traybake – the main ingredients of which are caster sugar and flour.[37] The more I read, the more confusing (yet also fascinating) it became. It was the discovery of the website created by the increasingly well-known Swedish 'Diet Doctor', Andreas Eenfeldt MD,[38] that just about tipped the balance in favour of considering an approach that went more in the low-carb direction.

I had one more thing on my side: I needed to lose a few kilos myself. My diet is very varied, albeit more savoury than sweet, and I now believe that this has played a role in why I have never shown any tendency to diabetes myself. That being said, my jeans waist size had steadily increased from 34 inches (twenty years ago) to 38 inches in 2012, and that was clearly not good. It didn't help that my preferred Levi's 501 jeans spell out your waist size on the outer label … and I was approaching 95 kilos. So, with my new-found knowledge, I decided to go to Katy with a challenge. 'Will you try one last weight-loss approach together with me before going to the surgeons?' My personal goal was to go below 90 kilos again and at least get back into my 36-inch waist jeans. As for Katy, without too much coercion, she accepted a 10 kilo challenge (that's 22 pounds or 1½ stone), but would only guarantee me her support – and enthusiasm – if it was clearly working after two weeks. We also agreed that a drop of 10 kilos meant losing at least two dress sizes, which in many ways proved to be a more relevant measuring stick for her needs. 'More choice at the shops,' she said, before asking: 'Where do I begin?' As for me – well, I thanked her for her trust and confidence. That's how we got started.

---

37   Diabetes UK, n.d.
38   www.dietdoctor.com

So what's this dietary approach called?

Now, terminology is everything – so I tried to come up with a name for the dietary approach that we would be taking. The closest I could come was LCHF (low-carb, high-fat), which is the expression that's been popularised in the Scandinavian countries. The Banting Diet represents a similar idea in South Africa. That latter approach is named after the first documented successful low-carb approach, which was made by the 'celebrity' undertaker, William Banting, in London during the 1850s (yes – successful 'low-carbing' has been going on for a long time). But, for Katy, I initially called it a 'modified Atkins diet'. This was so that if in doubt, she could easily read up or search online for more about the major success factors. It is well-documented that Dr Robert Atkins also read up on the history of dieting when facing his own weight issues in the late 1960s, and as a result personally focused on lowering his carb intake. His personal success with this approach would later become the inspiration for his bestselling book, *Dr Atkins' Diet Revolution,* originally published with remarkably little fanfare in 1972.[39] His focus was primarily on upping protein and fat levels, and he concentrated directly on weight loss, with less to say about the principles of healthy eating; but times were very different, and the latest version of his diet has moved on a bit. Incidentally, according to Wikipedia,[40] Dr Atkins died in April 2003, at the age of 72, after slipping on ice and hitting his head. Following that, he went into a coma. Before his death, while on life-support in hospital, he put on nearly 30 kilos because of fluid retention; a sad weight gain right at the end of his life.

The diet I would be proposing to Katy would have certain important differences from the essential low-carb principles; it included a greater focus on fresh vegetables and the elimination of seed oils such as soy,

39   Atkins, 1972.
40   Wikipedia, n.d. (1).

corn and sunflower. It would stress the importance of free-range eggs and organic butter – but other than that, it had many similarities.

Further reading, discussions with experts in the field and a later nutrition course which I followed (and passed) led me to my current convictions, which identify more closely with the hormonal effects of the different types and combinations of foods that we eat. But, back then, 'low-carbing' was my basic starting point. The low-carbohydrate principle is a simple one, and it stands out amongst the over-complication of many scientific explanations of bodily digestive processes. It goes like this: if you eat fewer carbs – that's starches and sugars – your blood sugar (glucose) level remains low and the resulting amount of insulin that your pancreas secretes is also limited. It is a principle that most diabetics are familiar with as they seek to balance blood sugar, also known as glucose and insulin levels, in their bloodstreams. Diabetes in both its forms is, after all, a disease of carbohydrate intolerance – in spite of it not usually being expressed in that way.[41] Insulin stimulates the conversion of glucose into fat. That's why type-2 diabetics are often overweight.

A minority of people seem to cope well with carbs, but a growing and significant number who eat today's high levels of carbohydrate, particularly sugar, will have bodies which over time become resistant to insulin. At that point, the pancreas tries to compensate for this overload by pumping out yet more insulin, leading to the deposit of yet more fat reserves on the body. As referenced earlier, I now know that this process also switches off another important hormone, leptin, which should be acting as your hunger suppressant but gets simply overwhelmed.

Now, as I mentioned, the reason that in the end the term 'a modified Atkins diet' became my code name for Katy and me getting started was mostly that information about the Atkins diet was easy to reference in books and online. I was no expert, and she might well want to look for guidance or simply additional meal ideas. But those 'modifications' to the diet that I referred to included the complete absence of processed food. In setting guidelines that would provide our basis for healthy eating over the long-term future, our focus was to be on vegetables,

---

41   See Accurso et al., 2008.

certain fruits (notably berries), dairy produce (including eggs), and small amounts of fish or meat. The latter could gradually increase in quantity after a few weeks. This was not to be a protein-rich diet, as Atkins is often referred to, but a fat-rich diet. After all, the Inuit tribes in Northern Canada and Greenland used to stay fighting fit for many months of the year on a diet of 90% fat. Furthermore, the use of real fats such as butter, coconut and olive oil was to be encouraged over the industrially produced seed oils from the likes of sunflower, soy and corn – as was the eating of nuts and avocados. And, contrary to what you might think, the naturally occurring carbohydrates and fibre in salads and vegetables such as courgettes, cauliflower and beans were going to be more than adequate to provide a solid base for the diet. Switching from milk to cream in coffee or desserts would reduce the impact of the natural sugars found in milk. This would further reduce carbohydrate levels as well as adding back taste. Sugar was off-limits, but a little cheese after a meal was just fine.

We got started. The first surprise was that it proved to be an exceptionally tasty diet; reducing starches such as rice, potatoes and bread was quite doable. Substituting spiralised courgettes for pasta was a great success (although only if we squeezed out the excess water). Dropping all sugar was more of a challenge, and learning to eat cheese with celery and small sliced carrots rather than crispbread[42] was harder than expected. But ... the kilos dropped off. Low-carb diets are reputed to have the effect of reducing the water storage in your body, so your weight on the scales can drop off quite quickly at the start. If true, that would initially just represent a change in the composition of your body – but your knees and ankles would already be saying 'thank you' for the reduced load. After just two weeks, Katy measured five centimetres less at the waist. However, it was the motivation to beat type-2 diabetes and have a broader choice of normal dress sizes that drove Katy to keep going against the odds and eventually lose a total of 20 kilos over the next six months. Christmas 2012 was a happy time for Katy and the

---

42   Over time, we both became creative at making low-carb almond flour and sesame seed crispbread!

whole family. This was, to all of us, an amazing achievement – and one that led her doctor to open his eyes very wide when he next saw her. Ironically, he was not particularly interested in her dietary approach; just that she'd successfully lost weight and reduced her type-2 danger signs. I guess it's simply the way doctors are trained, with much more time focused on curing ailments than supporting a healthier lifestyle in the first place. Interestingly, my own doctor marvels at my improved HDL (good cholesterol) markers and reduced triglyceride levels that have been registered over the last couple of years but also has little interest in how it has come about! Anyway, back to Katy – it's probably worth remembering that her GP had earlier pushed hard on the low-calorie, low-fat bandwagon; he may even have been somewhat irked by her success with this less orthodox approach – or maybe I'm reading too much into it!

As for me, I lost 7 kilos. My weight now fluctuates between 87 and 88 kilos depending on the day. I lost my 7 kilos over a three-month period, and had to cut right on back those glasses of red wine that I had previously enjoyed of an evening. Now, however, with my body used to its new set-point of just below 88 kilos, I can still enjoy a lower-carb lifestyle and comfortably drink my wine when I choose to. 'Set-point' is a phrase we will use several times in this book, because that represents the new anchor point which forms the basis for how your body (and in particular its hormonal levels) reacts within your future, slimmer and healthier self.

Now, this is where a certain amount of dietary personalisation comes in. Regarding weight loss, going low-carb seems to work for most people, but finding the right amount of carbs to eat and enabling you to remain at your new set-point can take time. It's best to start with a big cut-back if you want to seriously lose weight. Then, according to your body's needs, gradually bring back a certain quantity of carbohydrates – being very, very careful with sugar and bread, which are both carb-rich. Eating more fat is crucial to the success of this dietary approach. Yet funnily enough, that's where I have had the greatest problems in getting people to give it a go; so much so that I started a website called www.fatisourfriend.com to help build awareness and gather information. Unfortunately, the word for fat on your body is the same as that for the fat in butter and milk and nuts. Saturated fats such as butter have been demonised ever since Ancel Keys' landmark seven countries study was launched in 1958.[43] However, as we now know from the longer term analysis of these studies, eating fat doesn't bring on heart disease or make you fat;[44] it's the eating of carbohydrates, particularly sugar, which does that. Using a base of over 120,000 non-obese men and women across the US and following them from 1986 to 2006, research results showed that[45] weight gain was most strongly associated with the intake of potato chips (1.69 lb), potatoes (1.28 lb) and sugar-sweetened beverages (1.00 lb). Weight loss, on the other hand, was most associated with the eating of yoghurt (-0.82 lb), nuts (-0.57 lb) and fruit (-0.49 lb).

In late 2014, the American journal *Annals of Internal Medicine* even published a paper[46] which suggested that there is no evidence supporting the long-standing recommendation to limit saturated fat consumption. How long will it be before this message reaches us punters, sitting in the stands? It may well be that there are currently just too many doctors and academics with big reputations at stake to let that message roll without them putting up a protracted fight. A journalistic review of America's allegedly misguided dietary guidelines was published in the *British Medical Journal* in September of 2015. It stated:[47] '… the literature shows that the low-fat, high-carbohydrate diet has not produced better health for Americans since it was first introduced as official government policy in 1980'. But, yet again, the article had the so-called experts passionately disagreeing about the proper role of saturated fats and carbohydrates in your diet. In agreeing with the article's conclusions, Arne Astrup of the University of Copenhagen wrote that the committee developing the guidelines:[48] 'seems to be completely dissociated from the top-level

---

43   For more information on Ancel Keys and the Seven Countries Study,
     see www.sevencountriesstudy.com
44   Malhotra, 2013.
45   Mozaffarian et al., 2011.
46   Chowdhury et al., 2014.
47   Teicholz, 2014.
48   Astrup, quoted by Husten, 2015.

scientific community, and unaware of the most updated evidence'. However, representing more of an 'establishment' voice, David Katz of Yale University School of Medicine, went on record saying that:[49] 'the dietary guidelines report is excellent, and represents both the weight of evidence, and global consensus among experts'. I guess you just have to choose your experts! All I can say is that having read the different viewpoints and seen the results with Katy, my viewpoint comes down firmly on the side of those saying that fat has been much maligned for too many years and that our grandparents, who knew that sticky cakes and sweets were what added on the pounds, were quite right.

Another reason why fat in your diet is good for you is that it fills you up quickly, facilitating your body's uptake of vitamins and letting the 'I'm full' leptin response function properly. Propaganda – by which I refer to the official viewpoint as told by governments, such as that found in wartime posters of the 'Your Country Needs You' variety – has led to the current demonisation of fat. The latest guidelines provided by the 'eatwell plate', published by the British National Health Service, still lump fats together with sugar and request that you[50] 'avoid food and drinks high in fats and sugar'. When combined with processed carbs in a Snickers bar or a MacDonald's hamburger bun, I agree with them – but in those examples, we are discussing industrially prepared and highly processed junk food; another story entirely.

Let's take a real life example – my niece, Ellie. She wanted to lose 5 kilos but had previously only achieved such success on a highly disciplined juicer-diet, where she was limited to pre-prepared liquid drinks over a three-week period. The good news for her was that it had worked, and the dietary approach helped her squeeze into her wedding dress in which she looked svelte and beautiful. But, not surprisingly, that dietary approach provided no help when it came to keeping off the pounds that she had just lost. To be clear, I was not trying to force her onto a diet of any sort at the time, but she had seen my slimmed-down sister-in-law at her wedding and had naturally asked 'How did Katy go about it?'.

---

49   Brown, 2015.
50   NHS, 2014.

Apart from being something of a fussy eater, Ellie's real problem when considering this dietary approach was quite different. She was thirty years old and had thus grown up in the 'low-fat is good, cholesterol is bad' world, which still dominates to this day. When confronted with this new approach, she simply could not bring herself to drop the Flora ultra-light margarine and start eating butter, even though she admitted that it tasted much better. She said that she could taste the fat in fatty milk (as she called it) and she wasn't sure if she liked that either. I reminded her that it was actually natural whole milk we were talking about, but when it came to her low-fat cheese slices – well, to her, they were just obviously healthier than the full-fat (aka normal and less processed) cheddar that I wanted to put in front of her. Weren't they? Although Ellie bought in to the whole insulin story that I explained and to the role of leptin appetite suppressants (hers were clearly not functioning normally), she just felt that fat was not good for you and could not really accept such an approach. In a nutshell, the low-carb part sounded sensible but she couldn't get her head around the high-fat element. I do understand. If you've been told something is good for you and something else is a 'naughty pleasure' for your entire life, it's risky to break ranks.

The thing is: if you do decide to reduce carbs, they need to be replaced with something or you'll end up on a low-calorie yo-yo diet again. To satisfy your body's needs at a physical and also a hormonal level, eating more fat is important. Ellie's best friend, Kerry, did buy in to the new big picture and was prepared to give it a go. She became my next success story, losing a stone – just over 6 kilos – in two months. By accepting the 'fat is our friend' mantra and changing her cooking approach to include such things as toasting her own home-made granola and using cauliflower mash to replace potatoes in her favourite foods, she was slimming healthily. It's perhaps worth a quick mention here that these recipes are all available in the relevant section of the 'fatisourfriend' website.

What's still counter-intuitive to many, though, is that eating fat does not make you fat, but that eating carbohydrates in the form of bread, cakes and cereals does.[51] Remember: however healthy they try and make that pack of cereal flakes or crunchy muesli look, more than half of the content takes the form of highly processed carbohydrates that will spike your blood sugar, drive up your insulin levels, stimulate fat storage on your body and make you feel tired one or two hours after you have finished eating. One of the great reactions I get from people following a lower-carb, higher-fat diet is that they have more energy. This is sometimes expressed by the fact that they no longer feel tired mid-afternoon or no longer feel hungry mid-morning. Or, as with Katy's situation (did I mention this earlier?), she now delights in walking up the stairs at work.

It all comes down to the same thing. Some carbohydrate intake is surely good for you, but the world in which we now live has grown top-heavy in carbs. It's hard to get away from them. A Big-Mac meal consists of carbs in the burger bun, carbs in the fries and carbs in the Coke or Fanta, all supplemented with some fat and protein in the thin burgers. A large classic pizza from Pizza Hut is 60% carbohydrate by weight. Of the 73 grams of protein, fat and carbs in a Starbucks blueberry muffin, 55 of those grams are carbohydrates in the form of sugar and flour – that's a whopping 75%. Nevertheless, most journalists and medical researchers still refer to junk food diets as high in fat – simply because they consider the carbohydrates innocuous. In the 1970s, '80s and '90s, the nutritional studies that got funded and published almost all examined the various supposedly negative effects of eating fat – in particular, saturated fat. Very few considered the possible role that carbohydrates play in our fattening society. Since the turn of this century, sugar is again back in the limelight and research projects studying the effects of carbonated drinks are very much in vogue – but it's worth noting that the impact of wheat and other cereals still goes relatively un-studied! As recently as 2000, the American Heart Association[52] was encouraging you to eat 'gum-drops' and 'hard candies made primarily with sugar' to avoid eating those dreaded fatty foods.

---

51 Tenderich, 2012.
52 American Heart Association, 2000, p.22.

Summing up, there are only three macronutrients in the food you eat: fat, protein and carbohydrates. Today's conventional wisdom dictates that you eat most of your calories in the form of carbohydrates because of the alleged (but now largely disproven) link between dietary fat and heart disease. The only really bad fats appear to be those artificially made trans fats which used to be major constituents of margarine and seed-based cooking oils, but these are now being slowly legislated out of the picture. Yet since you can only eat so much protein (and if you are educated to believe that fat is harmful), you are left with carbs as your main source of food and energy. That has led so many well-intentioned people to give poor high-carb based dietary advice for so many years.

If you do want to change your body shape, have more energy and lose weight for the long-term, I'm pretty confident that you can manage it without too much difficulty when at home; but I admit you will have to work on how you adapt some of your routines in daily life. Lunchtime sandwiches, for example, are out – but a number of ideas for how you can cope with that are to be found later on in this book.

What really drives 'diabesity'?

Katy's problems, which she shares with many, are often summed up these days by the term 'diabesity'; an amalgam of the words 'diabetes' and 'obesity'. But what exactly does that mean, and what is causing the huge increase in numbers of those diagnosed with this malady? Diabesity is the term used to cover the full range of metabolic disturbances, from mild blood sugar and insulin imbalances to pre-diabetes and eventually full blown type-2 diabetes. It occurs in around 80% of overweight people, but it also occurs in about 40% of people of normal weight – those being the so-called 'skinny fat' people who look thin but are metabolically fat and have all the same risk factors for disease and death as those who are overweight. They manage to look slim – but only on the outside.

Although the word 'diabesity' is something of a catchphrase for a variety of sins, it needs to be taken very seriously. As a potentially deadly disease that more than one in three of us have today, it saps our energy, making us fat and ill – yet many of us don't even know we have it. It's all very well exhibiting the signs of mild insulin resistance, but – given the choice – you certainly don't want to experience type-2 diabetes.

Type-2 diabetes is a disease of carbohydrate intolerance, where your pancreas pumps out too much insulin simply because your diet is full of empty, carb-rich foods. These (usually highly processed) foods contain sugars and other starchy carbohydrates. You may be eating them in the form of bread, pasta, rice, pastries, cereals, cakes, chocolate or biscuits. Being carb-rich foods, they necessitate the secretion of higher quantities of insulin just to keep up with your body's attempts to balance out high blood sugar levels. This, in turn, starts a vicious cycle – the first sign of which is insulin resistance. Over time, this leads to energy loss and premature ageing while also being associated with diseases of the heart, cancer and dementia.

When that vicious cycle kicks in, you get hungry. You exhibit rising insulin levels, which make you even hungrier. However, your hormonal leptin doesn't function well; you don't feel full and so you eat more and put on weight, also causing inflammation and creating oxidative stress. Time-stressed doctors have little option but to treat your high blood sugar levels, whereas the real solution lies in reducing your levels of insulin. That's where a low-carbohydrate diet plays its critical role. Fortunately, insulin resistance and diabesity are usually completely reversible. Researchers at the Newcastle Magnetic Resonance Imaging Centre found that in people who had suffered from type-2 diabetes for four years or less, major weight loss returned insulin secretion to normal. A leaflet entitled *Reversing Type-2 Diabetes* is available at their website[53] (though it should be noted that they do not specifically recommend a low-carb, high-fat dietary approach). If you want to obtain more medical advice on the issues involved here from an experienced diabetes doctor's perspective, I can thoroughly recommend reading *Reverse Your Diabetes* by Dr David Cavan,[54] who is also an advocate of diet and lifestyle changes.

Weight gain, elevated blood sugar levels, high blood pressure and high levels of triglycerides and LDL (bad) cholesterol are among the typical early warning signs for diabesity. And, although there are certainly some genetic components, we can all improve our chances of avoidance through considering differently what we eat and drink and taking moderate levels of exercise.

From skeletons and tissue that have been analysed, both diabetes and obesity were extremely rare in hunter-gatherer cultures. Two recent studies have shown that a paleolithic-style diet (free of cereal grains, seed oils and excessive fructose) can produce dramatic improvements in both cardiovascular and metabolic markers. An initial study[55] by Dr Staffan Lindeberg (University of Lund, Sweden) and his colleagues, with twenty-nine people suffering from heart disease, showed weight reduction (particularly fat loss in the midsection), an improvement in glucose tolerance and a voluntary reduction in the absolute volume

---

53 Taylor, 2015.
54 Cavan, 2014.
55 Lindeberg et al., 2007.

of food being eaten. In other words, while losing weight, they were – importantly – not hungry.

In the research team's second (smaller, follow-up) trial,[56] with thirteen diabetic patients, the patients also all lost weight – with five of them getting off their medication completely. But eight out of the thirteen patients still had higher than average blood glucose levels. This reminds us that dietary interventions can be very helpful but cannot always reverse diabetes once the body's ability to secrete insulin is reduced. Putting this differently: the earlier you remove toxins such as sugary carbs from your diet, the better your body's ability to prevent and reverse diabesity.

After losing 20 kilos, Katy's blood markers are much improved. She's still taking medication for diabetes, albeit at a much lower strength than earlier. We will see how things progress. For now, let's take a look at a recent published case study from the *British Medical Journal* before moving on to Katy's successful dietary approach.

---

56   Jönsson et al., 2009.

Low-carb cure?
A case study on 'de-prescribing':
British Medical Journal, August 2015

Abbreviated and paraphrased from a case review published in the *British Medical Journal (BMJ).*[57]

The patient: A fifty-two-year-old man with a history of type-2 diabetes for fourteen years and hypertension for nine years presented to his general practitioner. He was a non-smoker with an alcohol intake of eight units a week. His problems: bloating, abdominal pains and erratic motions for over a year. He drove about twelve thousand miles a year for his job and found the loose motions 'a real worry'. His weight was 108.8kg (steady for ten years), BMI was 34.4, waist 113 cm, blood pressure 130/80 mm Hg (steady for some years).

He wondered whether any of his problems might be caused by his drugs and asked if he could cut down on any. He admitted to being afraid that his diabetic control might deteriorate and that he might need insulin, like some of his relatives.

Current Medication: Aspirin 75 mg once daily, Metformin 500 mg 3 times daily, Perindopril 4 mg daily, and Simvastatin 40 mg at night.

Diagnosis: Metabolic syndrome. Definitions vary but are based on insulin resistance, hypertension, obesity, and dyslipidaemia.

Recommendation: Arguably none of his drugs is essential – they have all been prescribed to reduce his risk of cardiovascular events and the complications of diabetes, not to treat an actual disease. These risks also depend on lifestyle choices such as diet, smoking and exercise.

Discussion: We suggest that, rather than prescribing drugs to patients, healthcare providers should try to explain the benefits and harms so that

---

57   Unwin and Tobin, 2015.

patients and clinicians can come to a shared decision. A recent review discusses possible processes for de-prescribing and argues that this should be patient-centred and evidence-based. Shared decisions also improve a patient's satisfaction with health services, and potentially with clinical outcomes.

Patient outcome: <u>The patient steadily lost a total of 16kg over seven months and successfully stopped all four prescribed drugs by adopting a low carbohydrate diet</u> – in his words: 'more a lifestyle than a diet'. The weight loss enabled him to exercise and take up yoga. He has come off sugar altogether and cut out bread, potatoes, pasta, cereals, and rice. This has led to greater consumption of green vegetables, eggs, full-fat Greek yoghurt and cheese. The weight loss has been maintained for a year, so he weighs less now than at any time in his adult life. The goal of coming off all drugs was achieved in a stepwise manner as he lost weight – first metformin, then perindopril, followed by simvastatin and aspirin. This weight loss has been matched by improvements in other parameters, including improved HDL cholesterol and lower triglycerides. His bowel problems and abdominal pains ceased within days of stopping metformin, his energy returned, and he now needs 1½ hours less sleep a day.

His summary? He feels 'just much younger again'.

PART 3
KATY'S DIET

Establishing rules for healthier living/eating

Staying healthy should not be that difficult. After all, our bodies were designed to function efficiently; it sounds like plain common sense to say that if you eat as much of your food prepared from fresh ingredients as you can and walk pretty regularly, your body will pick up all the right nutrients and stay healthy. Yet when, for example, things are concentrated for you (as in cartons of orange juice), the work goes out of the preparation and you get too much of the pure nutrients. You couldn't eat more than two large oranges, but it's easy to drink ten when they are ready-pressed. That adds up to a lot of sugar – or fructose, to be precise! But staying healthy has to do with other things too, so let's add in that you should probably leave your smartphone alone after an early dinner, switching it off beforehand to help your brain relax. This aids the passage of food along your digestive tract and gains you a longer, deeper sleep. Staying healthy is as simple as doing things like that, but we all know that it's not easy to do in our time-starved and highly connected world.

When you consider the way Katy managed things at this stage in her life, we need to get more precise – particularly when it comes to what she ate and how she went about it. To start at the beginning, your first task (if you choose to try the approach outlined in this book) will be to stop eating all processed foods and focus almost entirely on fresh ingredients. It may sound frightening or hugely impractical (or both, at first), and I know it won't be easy – but believe me when I say it that it won't mean spending all your spare time in the kitchen! That change alone will have a positive impact on your own stomach's biodiversity – that community of gut microbes, weighing in at over 1 kilo, which facilitates digestion and is more accurately known as your microbiome. Your whole digestive system will thank you for this change, and that is exactly where Katy got started. It also provided her with a first step in getting her food-related hormones functioning correctly again. The list of pre-prepared and highly processed junk foods is long and includes many items: from sandwiches made with today's ubiquitous quick-rise and virtually yeast-free bread; through burgers, hot dogs and chicken nuggets; to almost everything that's on sale at your local Starbucks or Costa. Again, don't worry – your coffee habit is safe, although the snack food surrounding it is off-limits. Sugar in one highly processed form or another is added to an estimated 80% of what's on sale in US supermarkets,[58] and there's no reason to think that this figure is very different in European countries. Invariably, sugar is also to be found everywhere snack foods are sold. The UK's independent consumer watchdog, *Which?* magazine, recently compared the nutritional value of sandwiches.[59] It found that three of those tested contained more than three teaspoons of sugar each. These were: 'posh' cheddar and pickle on artisan bread (from Pret), brie and bacon panini (from Caffe Nero) and Mexican chicken baguette (from Greggs). Three teaspoons is 12 grams of sugar; but add in all the carbs from the wheat and you'll see how these quick and easy lunchtime snacks can overload your system by driving up blood sugar levels, adding weight, sapping energy and … if you're not careful, easing your slow descent towards becoming a victim of type-2 diabetes.

Admittedly, if you dedicate a lot of time to it, you will find some healthier prepared foods. For most of us, however, it's simply too complicated to find our way through the numerous ingredients lists and identify all the different words used for sugar and all the untested and potentially disruptive additives and emulsifiers. This does not take into account the small quantities of modified wheat and corn extract that are to be found in so many of our daily processed foods. What can sometimes help is the gluten-free label, but many manufacturers add in extra varieties of carbohydrate in their search for taste and consistency, often increasing the total carb impact over the regular goods. Potato flour, when used, has a greater proportion of carbs than wheat flour – but you do at least skip the protein.

After this re-focus on fresh ingredients, it is up to you to decide how fast you want to go with your weight loss before deciding how low you

---

58 Ng et al., 2012.
59 *Which?* magazine, April 2015.

want to go with your carbs. The thing is: starches and sugars are not essential to human life. You don't absolutely need to eat carbs to exist. Want proof? The Canadian scientist Dr Vilhjalmur Stefansson lived for many years with the Inuit tribes – more often known as Eskimos – in the early part of the twentieth century. They are famous for going months living almost exclusively on fish and meat, and he joined them in their eating habits with no health problems suffered. Few people believed his story upon his return, so, together with a fellow explorer, he decided to carry out a no-carb dietary test for one year. The results of this fascinating study were published in 1930.[60] Stefansson's resulting health markers after one year eating fish and meat were described by the doctors examining him as excellent. Funnily enough, the only time he experienced any problems was when the level of fat in his diet was reduced by the consulting doctors.

Lowering your carbohydrate intake right down will not affect your general disposition or health – at least not in the way that removing fat or protein would. If you were to drop your fat or protein intake way down, you'd become very ill and after just a week important bodily functions would stop working. Dropping carbs leads your body to adapt to using stored fat reserves;[61] you begin to shed the pounds. So, it's up to you to choose which level of carb reduction is appropriate. You can choose either:

- 'How low can you go' – the ketogenic, ultra-low-carb approach that helps you lose weight more quickly; or, simply:

- 'Cut back on the carbs' – cutting out sugar and cereals, steadily easing back on carbs from potatoes and rice and getting energised.

With either approach, having stopped eating all processed food (that covers pre-prepared meals and packaged foods of all kinds), you will need to move on to the next step and cut out all cereals. This includes wheat, barley and oats (all of which happen to contain gluten)

60   McClellan and Du Bois, 1930.
61   Ketogenic Diet Resource, n.d.

as well as – of course – 100% carbs in the form of sugar. There will be no bread or morning Weetabix any more. If you are an American reader, a full one-third of the most popular US breakfast cereal, Honey Nut Cheerios, consists of sugar. So, I am sorry to say it, but that's another boxed product which goes straight to the top of the list of foods to be replaced.

Your diet will effectively morph into a healthy mix of many different vegetables combined with dairy, nuts, fish and meat – as many of these as possible prepared by your own hands. If you are not used to cooking from scratch, it's worth noting that the staff working at the supermarket fish and meat counters will prepare what you want to cook so that the fresh food is ready for you to just stick in the pan. That goes for filleting a piece of fish, which you can just pop in the frying pan, or preparing an impressive crown roast of lamb for the oven. Providing you with a service is what they have trained for so it may be easier than you think to avoid the ready-to-cook food aisles and go for the fresh counters where that personalised service is free.

> ### Anja's Cheesy Cauliflower Mash
>
> Ingredients:
> - 1 head of cauliflower.
> - 30g cream.
> - 20g butter.
> - 50g cream cheese.
> - 50g grated cheddar, gruyère or comté.
> - Salt and pepper to taste.
>
> Method:
> 1. Break up the cauliflower into smaller pieces.
> 2. Microwave (covered) with the cream, cream cheese and butter for 5 minutes. Stir well and continue for 5 further minutes.
> 3. Mix in the grated cheese and seasoning, then puree with a hand blender or mash well.
>
> Quick, delicious, low-carb and nutritious!

I have found that, for many, it is the thought of cutting out bread that can fill them with horror and be enough to stop them approaching this diet. This even includes some people with type-2 diabetes on the horizon. Bread is everywhere. You may also be thinking that it hits all the oh-so-practical, quick and convenient buttons. But don't worry; you won't miss it as much as you think, and there are some good, filling and nourishing replacements – but more of that later.

In traditional terms, we sometimes think of eating meat and two veg, with one of those veggie portions usually taking the form of mashed potatoes or chips, or maybe rice or pasta. As you move forward with this approach, you will be talking 'two real portions of veg' or 'three real veg', if you prefer. Imagine: cauliflower cheese and green beans accompanying your grilled chicken; Katy's stir-fry vegetables as a delicious dish by itself or with some similarly stir-fried beef with Chinese spices; or spaghetti bolognaise with grated/spiralised courgettes and carrots as the 'pasta' base.

Katy's Favourite Vegetable Stir-Fry

Ingredients:
- Prepare some chopped-up garlic, chilli, ginger and onions.
- Quarter a few mushrooms.
- Chop some mange-tout in half, diagonally.
- Wash and chop a handful of small pieces of broccoli.
- Have some soy sauce and sesame oil ready for taste, but use coconut oil or butter for frying (ghee is best).

Method:
1. Heat up a large saucepan or wok and add 1 tsp of coconut oil.
2. Put in the garlic, chilli, ginger and onions for a smoky-hot 10 seconds before adding all the other ingredients ... shake it about a bit!
3. After 3 minutes or so, drizzle on the soy and sesame oil for 1 further minute. Shake and serve.

It's ... you know it's ... quick, delicious, low-carb and nutritious!

It helps to think of your new lower-carb ingredients list as a tool kit to inspire you with exciting combinations such as cheesy cauliflower mash, ratatouille, moussaka, intense ragout sauces, bolognaise, roast rosemary chicken, smoked salmon slices with sour cream, chopped chives and hard boiled eggs, or your own delicious home-made mayo added to sliced cold cuts of roast beef and pork ... and so many more. Finish meals off with simple desserts such as small portions of fresh fruit, berries with cream, Greek yoghurt or a selection of cheeses together with your own home-made crispbread. There is also a host of low-carb desserts – ranging from sticky toffee pudding to custard – that can be made using artificial sweeteners, but my advice is to limit them to just once a week. It's less about the questionable nature of some artificial sweeteners than because many people find that the more sweetness you come across, the more you want. So it's best to first adapt to less sweetness by eating strawberries and cream without sugar, for example. Do this with a smile and see it as a form of personal training!

The specific approach that Katy followed was based on the fundamental guidelines of lowering carbohydrate levels and increasing intake of natural fats such as butter, lard, olive oil and coconut oil, while recognising the need for a healthy biodiversity in her stomach's bacterial digestive system. She decided to drop all rice and potatoes, too – although that way of eating still gave her a certain quantity of carbs from all the vegetables she ate; it's just that the daily proportions changed. Mashed potatoes are 15% carbs by weight, while mashed cauliflower with cream and cheese works out at less than 5% – and believe me, it tastes great. A slice of buttered toast contains about 15 grams of carbohydrate, while a cheese omelette has none at all.

So here is what worked for Katy:

1. **Drop all pre-prepared and processed food.**

2. **Drop the carbs ... say no to breads, potatoes, pasta, rice and sugar ... including pastries & cookies.**

3. **Get creative with all the other ingredients you can now use!**

Quantities? Side effects? Exceptions?

A word on how much you can eat. If you decide to take the 'How low can you go?' approach, as Katy did, it may well be because you have a lot of weight you want to lose. Remember, Katy's first major goal, which she achieved in two months, was to lose 10 kilos. Although you are not encouraged to do any substantial physical exercise during this phase (see page 98 for more info), you will need to exercise some portion control, and that will also means skipping all fruit at the start of this more intense approach. Don't worry; you'll get all the vitamins you need from the meat, fish and many different vegetables you eat – but there may be some side effects as your body switches to burning its fat reserves. You may at first experience cravings, particularly for sugar, as you embark on this journey. Headaches, fatigue and even a little light-headedness can occur at the start. But there is a simple fixer-upper, and that's to drink enriching bouillon made from a stock cube diluted in a cup of boiling water – get the organic variety if you are using store-bought stock cubes or make your own chicken stock. And drink lots of water.

Home-Made Chicken Nuggets

Ingredients:
- 2 small boneless chicken breasts (thigh meat tastes even better).
- 1 large egg.
- 3–4 tbs coconut oil for frying.
- 'Breadcrumbs':
- 3 parts ground pork rinds.
- 1 part almond flour.
- 1 part parmesan cheese.
- Salt and pepper to taste.

Method:
1. Grind up the pork rinds and mix with all the other ingredients except the egg.
2. Cut up the chicken into bite-sized pieces before putting it in the beaten egg and coating.
3. Cover each nugget with the dry 'breadcrumbs' before frying on all sides in the coconut oil until crisp and golden or roasting for 15 minutes in the oven at 200°C, turning once.

Some people like to count the grams of carbs in what they eat if they want to get to a really low level of carbohydrate intake, but generally I suggest simply using the low-carb checklist. It shouldn't be necessary to get too analytical here so it's best to learn to recognise what you can and can't eat, then get creative using some of the inspirational ideas in this chapter or on the website. Or you can just roam the internet for fresh insights.

Being creative can take you to unusual places, depending on your taste buds. Matt, a friend of mine with a few pounds to lose, ended up with a highly spiced approach, adding in garlic, ginger and chilli to much of what he eats. Katy, on the other hand, developed some even more unusual eating combinations at the time – her favourite being fried bacon and pickled gherkins (and no, she wasn't pregnant!). She still loves to eat another diet speciality each week – fried or poached salmon served with fresh tzatziki. However you decide to go about it with this new 'tool-kit' of ingredients, you should never go hungry. As your insulin/leptin receptors return to normal (and as long as there is enough fat in your diet) you will feel full more quickly than you are used to. Your body adapts quite quickly.

If you initially struggle with those sweet cravings, although sugar substitutes should be only used occasionally, this might be where you want to make an exception and go for some sugar-free jelly with whipped cream. You're transitioning, after all! The exception proves the rule and even a couple of squares of 85% dark chocolate are allowed. I know; you're probably used to Cadbury or something similar but more than a half of Dairy Milk chocolate is in fact sugar (56%) – much more if you buy the US version. For a product to be called chocolate in Europe, at least 30% of the ingredients by weight must be chocolate (cocoa powder and solids) – but read the label of Cadbury Dairy Milk and you will find it is carefully worded as 'family milk chocolate'. As such, it is allowed to contain just 20% cocoa.[62] In the US, that minimum is set at just 10% –

---

62   Metz, 2015.

but although the step up to 85% may take some getting used to, it can be done and is even associated with some heart benefits.[63]

Katy cut out all fruit, but began to eat small portions of berries and whipped cream once she'd dropped 10 kilos. During the next four months, she steadily lost further weight before stabilising at just below 80 kilos – a full 20 kilos lighter than at the start of the diet. She's still pleasantly plump (her words, not mine) because she decided to stabilise at that level – but her doctor is much happier, her blood sugar levels are improved and she thrives on having a lot more energy.

---

63   Djousse et al., 2010.

Going low-carb: Getting started, step by step

My recommendation is that you work your way into this way of eating for a week or so, steadily adapting to a low-carb, high-fat diet – or rather, to this new way of life. Because that is what it will become. There is no point in adapting for ten weeks, improving your blood markers and successfully losing weight before simply returning to a standard Western diet. Don't let this thought alarm you, though, because in the future you will still be able to make exceptions – even the occasional binge will do you no long-term harm – but you will never be able to return 100% to the over-carbed, over-processed junk food diet that rules today. Our society thrives on providing you with carbohydrate-based snack and junk foods of all kinds, and to change that, you will need to sort out your life accordingly. You may remember that in the long-term survey of 120,000 women and men published in the *New England Journal of Medicine* in 2011,[64] the greatest weight gains over twenty years were correlated with the consumption of potato crisps/chips.

One thing is clear: every life situation is unique, and how you go about change will be unique to you and your situation. Katy was working in a school where the canteen always offered up fresh salads – and there was a choice of cooked veggies too! Lucky her. Kerry, who this summer is currently following the same low-carb approach, loves to make jam-jar salads with the dressing at the bottom – a quick shake and she's ready for lunch. Alex, a fussy eater who just wanted to eat more healthily, prepares large quantities of his meat and vegetable ragout sauce and pre-mixes it with different vegetables before freezing it in portion-sized poly-bags and then microwaving it at the Internet start-up company where he works. You just need to plan your days ahead a little and take control of your lifestyle ... but I'm afraid sandwiches and hot-dogs are definitely on the 'No' list!

---

64   Mozaffarian et al., 2011.

Your introductory week:

It is best to get started by steadily reducing the proportion of carbs (sugars and starches) in your diet and replacing them with more vegetables (a preference goes to those growing above the ground, which are lower in carbs), nuts, berries, meat and seafood. You can try going cold-turkey, but doing things this way helps acquaint you with what carbs are, how you can spot them and how you will go about avoiding them in future.

Next, clear out the cupboard of all tempting delicacies. Whether it's a bag of crisps, a box of corn flakes, a bar of milk chocolate, some digestive biscuits, or (worst of all) sugar-rich energy bars ... you'll need to remove them to help you fight any lingering carb temptation. You shouldn't feel the need to snack too much between meals in the future, but olives, nuts and sticks of celery dipped in cream cheese will present you with some new and healthy opportunities. You've been eating the way you do for years, so it's not surprising that you'll miss a few things at first. Prepare to create a new balance in your meals, and accept that what's on your plate will sometimes look a bit different! Eating 'spaghetti' bolognaise made with drained courgette (zucchini) or squash noodles may at first sound like a turn-off, but you'll be surprised at how good they taste!

It's time to get started:

Stop eating bread, wheat-based cakes and all pastries.

Reduce any added sugar in stages until it's mostly just there in fresh fruit – when you eat it.

Avoid all highly processed foods, including fast food and anything labelled 'low-fat' or 'low cholesterol'.

Start eating your fat and protein, whether it is meat, fish, cheese or eggs, together with your favourite selection of fresh vegetables, or a mixed salad.

As a good basic guide, those vegetables growing above the ground (such as cauliflower, beans, courgettes and aubergines) are lower in carbs than root vegetables – so potatoes, which are (strictly speaking) tubers, should not be eaten at all or should be limited to use as a small, salad ingredient. Turnips are not allowed, at least while you are going really low in carbs, although turnip tops (the greens that grow above the ground and which you can steam or boil up) are absolutely fine to eat. The same logic applies to beetroots, parsnips and turnips – at least until you are well-entrenched in the diet. These root vegetables are rich in nutrients, but you'll have to skip them for a while. On the other hand, sauces made with butter, with thick, sugar-free Greek yoghurt or with cream are to be welcomed … even encouraged. It might all seem a bit counter-intuitive – at least until you get used to things.

The simple truth is that there are many home-made, easy-to-prepare recipes using basic staple ingredients and fresh meats and vegetables that are much, much healthier for you than what the food industry has prepared and packaged. And, when it comes to fat, you should avoid oils like margarine or canola oil that still contain small amounts of trans fats and are largely made from seed oil. You should also avoid liquid versions of those industrially produced seed oils such as sunflower, safflower, soybean and corn oil. They are overly rich in omega-6, which we get more than enough of in our Westernised diets, and which contributes to inflammation – as you will have read earlier. Cook and drizzle with healthy oils such as olive oil – or organic rapeseed if you like the taste. Use dairy butter and its close relation, ghee (a form of clarified butter) when cooking. Both of these are good for you, as are all saturated fats – including lard, beef dripping, goose fat, any duck fat you may have left over after frying a duck breast and (of course) coconut oil. Using palm oil is also a good thing as long as you are sure of its provenance – a lot of environmental damage has been attributed to the recent expansion of plantations.

Weights and quantities – how much can I eat?

There's no reason to be too analytical here. Some 'low-carbers' weigh and measure everything they eat, but Katy's experience shows that this is not necessary. What you will be able to do quite quickly is simply recognise what you can and can't eat, just as you will learn to recognise that fresh fruit is much healthier for you and less sugary than squeezed juice … then you can be creative in how you go about using your ingredients. There are many ideas in this chapter and on the website to get you started. If you choose to maximise weight loss and reduce carbs as much as you can, I suggest you use the more restrictive 'How low can you go' list as your guide. Over a few days, that will take you to the fastest fat-burning phase, where your liver is producing ketones to complement and replace the glucose your brain and body needs. More about that in the section called 'Going ketogenic' on page 108.

Your basic low-carb checklist:

There's no reason to be too analytical here; it is much more important to develop the ability to recognise what you can and can't safely eat – then you can mix and match and get creative. Some people count the individual grams of carbs when they want to go really low-carb – but I suggest simply using the more restrictive 'How low can you go' list as your guide in the 'Going ketogenic' section on page 108.

VEGETABLES	
(including fruit with lower sugar levels such as tomatoes)	
Smaller portions please	**Best for you**
Avocados	Cauliflower (also grated for faux risotto)
Tomatoes	Greens such as cabbage, Brussels sprouts, kale (of course!), spinach, turnip tops, etc.
Red, green and yellow peppers	Cucumber, celery, lettuce, radishes, arugula

Onions and garlic	Broccoli
Peas	Okra
Canned pinto beans	Courgettes (zucchini) and marrow – try spiralising
Boiled beetroot (in small quantities)	Eggplant (aubergines)
	Green beans
	Mushrooms
	Spaghetti squash
	Chicory (and chicory roots)
	Asparagus

All these vegetables are great fresh, but sometimes growing seasons are short, so frozen is fine too. Just as long as you check that you're buying the pure vegetable and not a ready-made blend such as red cabbage and apples or spinach pre-mixed for Greek dishes etc.

DAIRY	
Good for you	**Best for you**
Milk (whole milk) in limited quantities	Cream
All hard cheeses; also camembert and brie	Aged cheeses – best from raw milk – such as parmesan, comté and camembert
Cottage cheese, cream cheese and ricotta	Soft goats' milk cheeses
Yoghurt (only plain)	Greek or other strained yoghurts (straining gives a higher fat content)
Butter	Butter from pastured cattle
Eggs	Eggs from free-range chickens with a varied diet

FRUIT	
(only one hand-sized piece or a small handful of berries per day)	
Good for you	**Best for you**
Apples and pears	Berries such as strawberries, raspberries, blackberries, etc.
Plums	Cherries
Melons in general	Watermelon
Apricots and peaches	Nectarines
Grapes	

MEAT	
Good for you	**Best for you**
Chicken breast	Chicken drumsticks from free-range sources
Pork tenderloin	Pork chops (best from free-range sources)
Beef – such as roast beef	Beef from grass-fed cattle
Liver pate – pork, chicken or fowl-based	Make your own chicken liver pate
Bacon and salami	Bacon and salami from artisan and free-range sources
Lamb	Liver, kidneys and other offal
Minced pork, beef and lamb (veal also available in many European countries)	The best quality you can afford – but never take the lower-fat option

NUTS and other tasty morsels (here you'll need to use 30 grams as a measure)	
Good for you	**Best for you**
Cashews (not so low-carb – so 10 in a portion)	Walnuts and pecans
Peanuts	Macadamia
Brazil nuts	Hazelnuts
Mixed nuts – salted is OK	Almonds – 25 or so in a portion
	Crispy kale chips (surprisingly tasty!)
	Home-made seed crackers

DRINKS (drink lots of still water)	
Good for you	**Best for you**
Dry white wine (limited quantities)	Dry red wine (limited quantities)
Belgian beer (once a week!)	Iced tea (unsweetened; squeeze of lemon)
Iced tea (use some sweetener if you need to)	Kombucha (unsweetened)
Sparkling water	Coffee (with cream but no sugar)
Tomato/carrot/kale juice (check for the best ingredients)	Regular tea and infusions (tisanes)
	Herb teas and fruit infusions
… No fruit juices, except a teaspoon of lemon or lime for flavouring water	

FISH	
Good for you	**Best for you**
All fish	Oily fish such as mackerel, salmon, sardines and tuna
Prawns, shrimp, crayfish, etc.	Organic or similar
Mussels, oysters and all other shellfish	
Lobster	

More advice ...

WHAT MUST BE AVOIDED!	
Bad for you	**Worse**
All pre-prepared foods and drinks	
All vegetable seed oils	
All cereal-based foods; from Weetabix to bread ...	... particularly wheat when made into industrial breads and rolls
All low-fat products	
Take-aways; there are more carbs (especially sugar) than you think	

WHICH OILS AND FATS TO USE?	
Good for you	**Not recommended**
Lard	Sunflower and safflower
Duck and goose fat	Corn, peanut and soy
Butter (ghee is best for frying)	
Extra-virgin coconut oil	
Olive oil	
Organic rapeseed oil	

USEFUL BAKING AND COOKING RESOURCES	
Good for you	**And why …**
Almond flour	Much lower in carbs than wheat flour
Coconut flour	Lower in carbs than wheat flour; lots of fibre
Chia seeds	To add bulk
Psyllium husks	To thicken and add fibre
Shirataki noodles	Low-carb – but not to everyone's taste
Stevia as a sweetener – only when needed	
Erythritol sweetener (in moderation) if you don't like that Stevia aftertaste – only when needed	

Reading the food labels

Inevitably, even if you are using as many fresh ingredients as you can, there'll be a few store-bought staples which you just can't avoid using. How do you tell if they are low-carb enough for your purposes? Generally, using the information on the label about how many carbs can be found in 100 grams is the easiest way. It allows you to work out a simple percentage for easier comparison. You will need to subtract the fibre content if you are in the USA, but in Europe the carbohydrate reading is a net value; the assumption is made that the fibre will simply pass right through you! So … suppose you want to prepare a home-made dip to go with your home-made low-carb crackers. You consider making houmous. In its simplest form, that's just pureed chickpeas with a little garlic, lemon juice and olive oil, and you have a can of chickpeas in the cupboard. The oil you use contains no carbs by definition (fat is your friend, after all), and although lemon juice and garlic contain some, the quantities are small – particularly since you'll be sharing with a couple of friends. In deciding whether to go ahead, it all comes down to the chickpeas – so you get out your magnifying glass and examine the label. It looks something like this:

Canned chickpeas		
Nutritional value	**Per 100gms**	**Your thoughts as you read this info …**
Calories or kcal Energy Kj	139 587	I don't take into account the number of calories or kilojoules.
Protein	7.0	There's more than enough protein in what I eat, so I'm OK, thanks.
Carbohydrate … of which sugar	23.1 0.9	Not much 'quick-burning' sugar, which is good – but a net carb weight of (23.1 – 5.3 of fibre) = 17.8, which is still quite high.

Fibre	5.3	Good to know; healthy digestion.
Fat … of which saturated	0.9 0.0	I'm going to be adding some extra-virgin olive oil, which will dial this value up.

Considering that it's easy to demolish 100 grams per person of tasty houmous, you'll have to be careful if you do decide to go ahead with your plans – even when you are dipping with low-carb crackers, carrots and celery. Generally, net carb levels above 10% are considered high, so I would advise you to use that as a useful benchmark indicator. Given the choice, then, if you've time to roast an aubergine and then make that other tasty Middle Eastern delight, baba ghanoush, you'll do better; cooked aubergines have a net carb weight of just 7g/100g (7%). Or, you could try Annick's smoked salmon dip. She's a former colleague who now eats low-carb simply because she feels better that way. Pureeing all the ingredients together makes a smooth dip, if you prefer that – but my guests seem to like it when it contains small pieces of salmon. Taramasalata and that quick-to-make standby, guacamole, provide other low-carb dipping opportunities; usually being around 5-6% carbs – but check there are not too many additives if you run out of time and buy ready-made from the deli counter.

Anne's Low-Carb Eggy-Cheese Buns

The convenience of bread is that it forms a nice barrier to your fingers and stops the inside of a sandwich from making your hands all sticky! This gives you a practical equivalent, a sandwich ersatz that's egg- and cheese-based using chia seeds and psyllium husk (you'll probably need to get that at the health food store) to provide bulk and texture. These buns are perfect for any low-carb sandwich, such as a bacon sarny, or as a base for your eggs benedict.

Makes 4-8 buns according to size.

Ingredients:
- 4 eggs.
- 100g cream cheese.
- 100g grated cheddar, gruyère or comté.
- 10g psyllium husk.
- 20g chia seeds.
- 2 tsp baking powder.
- Salt, paprika and pepper to taste.

Method:
1. Beat eggs in your blender until they are smooth and fluffy.
2. Slowly mix in the cream cheese.
3. Stir in the dry ingredients.
4. Let the chia seeds and psyllium husk swell for about 20 minutes.
5. Spread out in 4-8 flat rounds on a baking sheet/tray and bake in the middle of a 200°C oven for 12-15 minutes until nice and golden.
6. Let cool before serving. Serve lightly toasted if preferred.

Meal ideas to get you started on high-fat, low-carbing

Now, while this is not a recipe book, these examples should give you ideas and help you get started on your own personal low-carb, high-fat diet. Remember: the principle is to first get used to eating this way before you start using the really low-carb options ... and then only if your aim is quicker weight loss.

Breakfast: First, do I have to eat breakfast?

Although nutritionists love to tell you how important it is, it's not. It really is up to you. According to food historian Caroline Yeldham,[65] the Romans didn't really eat it, usually consuming only one meal a day around noon – so go Roman if you want to. Another thing – fasting is generally seen as being good for your body, so if your 'fasting through the night' extends to when you are next hungry, which may be the following lunchtime, that's fine.

Hot breakfast: Can I eat a full English?

Yes! Well, almost; you'll have to skip the toast and go easy on the beans – but the fried egg, tomatoes, mushrooms, bacon and sausage (as long as it's mostly meat!) are all just fine, as is a slice of black pudding if it's to your taste. Mind you, your cuppa must be made with the tiniest drop of milk or some cream. Milk contains just under 5 grams of sugar (in the form of lactose) per 100 grams, with whole milk having fewer carbs than skimmed. Cream, however, usually has less than 2 grams ... and it all adds up.

Try eggs any way: poaching (it's easier than you think); slow-cooking your scrambled eggs with butter; or maybe cooking a three-egg cheese omelette if you're hungry. Like your eggs more sophisticated? Eggs benedict on low-carb cheesy buns or a bed of spinach for eggs florentine

---

65   Quoted by Winterman, 2012.

are just some of the endless variations. My friend, Matt, goes for two soft-boiled eggs; peeled, put in a glass and mashed up with some salt and pepper. He tells me that in Germany they refer to that as a philosophers' breakfast! Even better when you dunk with some al dente asparagus spears ...

James' Low-Carb Granola ~ 1 kilo

Overview:

Mix your low-carb selection of nuts and seeds before toasting them on a tray in the oven for 30 minutes. Wait until you have just the right golden colours and then let the tray cool down with the oven door open.

Toasting Ingredients:

- 100g oats.
- 100g chopped pecans/walnuts.
- 150g blanched almonds, chopped or flaked.
- 50g hemp seeds, ground roughly.
- 100g flakes of coconut (no added sugar) ~ stir in after 15 minutes; they brown more quickly.
- 50g maple syrup.
- 100g water.

- 150g chopped hazelnuts.
- 50g sunflower seeds.
- 50g pumpkin seeds.
- 50g flax seeds.

- 75g coconut oil.

To serve: I add a few (5g) mixed raisins, currants or cranberries, or chop up a couple of fresh berries instead.

Method:

It's simple and quick, and making 1 kilo like this should keep you going for ages ~ unless you give some to your friends!

1. Chop the nuts and mix with the other toasting ingredients and with the maple syrup, coconut oil and water. Lay them out in an oven tray for roasting at 160°C for 15 minutes.
2. Give them a good mix, add the coconut flakes and return to the oven for another 10-15 minutes. It's that easy.
3. Leave to cool before storing for up to a month in an air-tight container. This balanced recipe gives 40 portions at 25 grams per portion (4 net grams of carbs). You can reduce this by dropping the oats (which I quite like for their consistency) and adding more nuts.

What about a cold breakfast?

Say no to cereal. When you eat conventional, carb-rich cereal, you put the flakes in the bowl and then add milk. Get used to putting yoghurt in your bowl and adding a few teaspoons of granola or berries as a topping. As for the type of yoghurt: Greek is best, being higher in fat and lower in carbs; just make sure it's full-fat. Avoid any flavoured yoghurts, whether Greek or not – they are inevitably sweetened with sugar or artificial sweeteners.

Granola is very popular in the US but less so in the UK and Europe. It comes from the word 'Granula', which was the world's first ever manufactured breakfast cereal, according to Wikipedia.[66] Because Mr John Harvey Kellogg was sued for using the word 'Granula', we have him to thank for the variant on the name that he registered, namely 'Granola'. This is now used generically to describe a kind of toasted muesli which, thanks to clever advertising and a fear of saturated fat and cholesterol which got eggs and bacon banned from the breakfast table, is generally thought to be very healthy. Except that it isn't, because of the sugar and the processed carbs.

Why make your own granola? First, it doesn't take long to make and the kitchen smells great while you are preparing it. More importantly, it's easy to get your home-made granola below 20% carbs by weight, whereas almost all store-bought versions are 50% carbs or substantially more. Jordans, as the UK market leader, recently celebrated their fortieth anniversary of selling granola in Britain. Bill Jordan, a British rock drummer, had been travelling round California and was inspired by what he'd eaten there. He launched Crunchy G when he returned to the UK. (It's since been renamed as Jordans Crunchy Oat.) To this day, it remains the brand leader in Britain, with over 40% of the granola market. Crunchy Oat Granola hits our breakfast tables with 64% carbs by weight – nearly half of them being from sugar. You will by now understand why, if you have decided to eat this way, it's banned from your breakfast table!

---

66   Wikipedia, n.d. (2).

To make commercial muesli and granola affordable and to please the UK's supposedly sweet tooth, it helps that oats, wheat and sugar are a relatively cheap source of carbs. The mixed nuts and seeds you'll be using if you make your own do cost a bit more, but I promise you, it's worth it. If you just fill yourself up with store-bought, processed muesli or granola, it will leave you with an energy gap mid-morning. That doesn't happen with slow-burning 'fatty' Greek yoghurt and your personal blend of toasted nuts, seeds and just a little fruit.

Meals: Try some comfort foods

Everyone likes shepherd's pie (or cottage pie if made with beef mince), but make it yourself using my recipe and it will give you an energy and vitamin boost. Try first substituting 50% cauliflower mash (mixed with potato) before going all the way to maximise your carb-reduction.

Meatloaf – it's an American classic, but is not made so often in the UK and Europe. You don't need flour or potato to hold it together – just a little egg – and it's quick and easy to make. Serve with your home-made tomato sauce and slice up what's left over for future use (or freeze).

Meatballs – another tasty low carb opportunity; add a little almond flour and egg to bind them, or try cooking them just as they are, rolled up and spiced with your favourite flavours.

Low-carb shrimp or crab cakes – use egg and a little almond flour to bind them together as they cook.

Hamburgers – use Anne's cheesy buns to replace the processed bread rolls, or go naked and just wrap with salad leaves – you're lowering carbs and eating healthily!

Chicken nuggets – yes, you can make your own from ready-minced chicken, or you can ask your butcher to prepare some. Add some finely diced onions and a hint of maple syrup for flavour, but skip the flour – it's unnecessary. A little egg wash and then finely grated parmesan cheese will give you a crispy exterior too. Alternatively, use pieces of chicken coated in my pork rind 'breadcrumbs'.

Stir-fried meat and veg – Chinese style, Korean or Middle Eastern; stir-fries are fresh and tasty and quick to make after a little prep work.

There are many options, and all the above-the-ground vegetables make excellent choices. Try serving with Pierre's egg-fried faux-rice.

Spiralised courgettes — spiralise or thinly slice courgettes before salting them to extract water and squeezing them in a tea-towel to get rid of the excess water. Then use them, raw or lightly fried, instead of pasta noodles with bolognaise, carbonara, vongole or your very own favourite pasta sauce. One word of caution: for the first ten days, go easy with pureed tomato sauces as they are quite rich in natural sugars. Tomatoes are, after all, really a fruit.

Salads:

Tuna salad — simply from a tin/can. Mix with finely chopped celery and/or cucumber before adding some almond flakes to add crunch. Add some home-made mayo, a dash of cream, and salt and pepper to taste. It's delicious.

Roquefort blue cheese, chicory and walnuts make an excellent combination but you can try salads of all sorts with

---

Pierre's Egg-Fried 'Faux' Rice

Ingredients:
- 1 cauliflower.
- 3–4 slices chopped bacon.
- 2 thinly sliced spring onions.
- 2 tbs coconut oil.
- 1 tbs each of fish sauce, soy sauce, and sesame oil.
- 1 tsp each of minced garlic and ginger.
- Squeeze of lime juice.
- 2 large eggs.
- Salt and pepper to taste.

Method:
1. 'Rice' the cauliflower florets in a food processor, or grate them.
2. Chop the bacon and spring onions.
3. Fry the bacon until very crisp. Then remove and set aside.
4. Add the coconut oil and gently fry the 'riced' cauliflower for 3 minutes.
5. Add and fry your garlic, ginger and spring onions at the side of the pan for 2 minutes.
6. Add the fish sauce, soy sauce, sesame oil, salt and pepper.
7. Mix together, adding your lightly mixed eggs and cook for a further minute.
8. Add your lime juice, bacon and any finely chopped left-overs of pork, chicken or shrimp.
9. Heat through for a perfect mock-rice dish.

some minor adaptations where needed. Caesar salad with nuts instead of croutons makes a good choice. Or why not prepare a lunch jar to shake and serve when needed? There are many more ideas at the fatisourfriend. com website.

Soups:

Soups are filling and nourishing. Try gently frying up a few diced onions, celery and carrots in a tablespoon of olive oil until soft before adding organic chicken or vegetable stock for extra flavour and diced courgette to add consistency. Add salt, pepper and a little chilli powder if you like. Then puree for a quick and easy vegetable soup which you can warm up at work for lunch on the next day.

Something special?

You can impress with low-carb cookery if you have the time and the inclination. Making a cheese soufflé using coconut flour as a low-carb but high-fibre thickener adds just a little intriguing flavour to a great low-carb dish – and it's surprisingly easy to make once you have the hang of it. Serve fresh from the oven for maximum effect.

Dessert:

Enter, once again, our friendly Greek yoghurt with berries – mixed with a dash of sugar ersatz, such as Erythritol, Stevia or even Splenda if your sweet tooth can't quite take the lack of a sugar sensation (absolutely no sugar, though).

Your cheese selection can range from relatively bland soft cream cheeses to the most pungent French munster cheese, though harder older cheeses are best in the early days of your diet. Let your taste buds roam but just make sure you are eating them with low-carb crackers or maybe a selection of raw vegetables.

Sammy's Low-Carb Crackers

These sound more complicated to make than they are, largely because you need to roll them out between two pieces of ovenproof parchment paper. Once you've made them once, it'll be easy! Use them for dipping or with smoked salmon or cheese.

Ingredients:
- 250g almond flour.
- 100g sunflower seeds, coarsely ground.
- 100g pumpkin seeds, coarsely ground.
- 100g sesame seeds.
- 100g ground quinoa/oats (omit for lowest carb content).
- 150ml boiling water.
- 50ml coconut oil.
- Pinch of salt.

Method:
1. Mix all dry ingredients lightly together before stirring in the boiling water and oil. Divide into two or three parts.
2. Spread the 'dough' onto one oven tray covered with baking paper; roll it thin (down to 3mm or roughly 1/8 inch) by placing an additional sheet of baking paper on top.
3. Roast/toast at 180°C for around 25 minutes or until golden brown, turning once.
4. When just out of the oven, sprinkle with a little salt and pepper.
5. Cool. Keep dry; they'll stay crisp for a few weeks.

Two 10g crackers have 2 net carbs, or just 1 net carb if you don't add in the quinoa/oats.

A Word on Digestion

Yes, digestion. In small quantities, you should have no problems, but some people (particularly those used to a diet rich in processed foods and breads) may well initially experience rumbling tummies and even minor discomfort if they eat lots of these — which you might, because they taste so yummy.

Snacks:

Eating fat-rich meals should leave you without the feeling that you need to snack very often. There are many options if you need to, though:

Nuts – almonds, hazelnuts, macadamia and walnuts are best, and it's fine to have them toasted with salt. (As a guideline, one portion is twenty-five or so almonds, but no more than ten cashews – they are relatively carb-rich.)

Dips – cream cheese by itself or mixed up with chopped herbs is perfect. Try Annick's smoked salmon dip using celery and/or carrot sticks, or even asparagus that's been boiled for just one minute, ready for dipping in Greek yoghurt or a soft-boiled egg. Guacamole and taramasalata make good choices, but be careful with houmous, which is good and healthy but relatively high in carbs.

Annick's Smoked Salmon Dip

A tasty low-carb dip that's fast to prepare.

Ingredients:
- 50g smoked salmon.
- 150g cream cheese.
- 20g cream.
- Chopped dill and spring onions.
- Salt and pepper to taste.
- 20ml olive oil.
- Juice of half a lemon.

Method:
1. Chop up the smoked salmon into small pieces.
2. Chop up the dill and spring onion.
3. Mix all the ingredients together.
4. Start dipping, preferably with Sammy's low-carb crackers.

Parmesan crisps – OK, they take a bit of time to make, but they are tasty and so 'moreish' that you must set some aside for the next day! Oh – and they're zero-carb.

Make your own low-carb home-made crackers, like Sammy does – they are the best! And what better than to dip the crackers in but your very own home-made baba ghanoush, Annick's dip or some home-made guacamole.

Chocolate – eating a couple of pieces is OK; even good for you. It has to be real, 85% chocolate though; anything less and it's too high in sugar.

Boiled eggs – eat them with ham and a little mayo if you like. You can, of course, use them mostly in salads such as Kathryn's Salad Niçoise on page 116, but they make a great, filling snack on their own and contain practically no carbs at all.

Drinks:

Only the low-carb alcoholic drinks like dry wines and sherry or the occasional spirit mixed with diet tonic are permitted (try and keep artificial sweeteners to a minimum, though). This rule isn't just about the carbs; because alcohol provides energy too, it is chosen by the body to be used as an energy resource before fat and protein – so drinking alcoholic drinks will slow you down if you're trying to lose weight.

Beer should be drunk only as a very occasional treat; try and make it a Belgian Trappist beer or something equally artisanal that will feed the flora of your digestive system. In this context, Professor Tim Spector of King's College London highly recommends it.[67] **Author's note:** such craft beers make an occasional treat later on in the diet, but they are too high-carb near the start if your focus is on losing weight!

Coffee is fine, but if you enjoy your cappuccino, you'll need to make it yourself because frothing cream diluted with water is the only low-carb way to go. Best to add a tablespoon of cream to your coffee – that's only about half a gram of carbs ... if you're counting them, that is.

---

67 In Spector, 2015, Chapter 15: *Contains Alcohol.*

Health Booster 1: Exercise

Yes – a brisk walk every day for fifteen minutes or so will help aspects of your muscular structure, increase the amount of protein and dietary fat that you process, aid your digestion, do wonders for your respiratory system and act as a pick-me-up for your brain by stimulating the flow of blood. If you want to do some gentle stretching exercises or yoga moves too, so much the better – this can help with IBS (irritable bowel syndrome) too.

But, unless you are taking it to athletic extremes, more strenuous aerobic exercise might (rather ironically) make you fat.[68] Running for long periods leads to muscle loss. This can, in turn, go on to affect your metabolism. When you run, your heart is usually working at a rate of two-thirds or more of its maximum capacity. As the length of exercise time increases, your body will go into a 'catabolic state', in which it begins to preserve its fat resources. Your 'old brain', which is responsible for fight or flight, begins to think that something is wrong with so many resources in use, so you start using muscle as fuel.

This leaves you with the situation that instead of burning up fat, longer runs slow down the process. You also begin to create stress hormones such as cortisol and adrenalin which encourage the body to store fat – so although (in the classical sense) you are 'burning' up a lot of calories, your appetite will increase, which may well put you right back where you started. No-one denies you will be a fitter person, but you probably didn't set out to also become a fatter person. In the words of Dr Richard Cooper and Dr Amy Luke of Loyola University Chicago's Stritch School of Medicine (who have both studied the connection between exercise and obesity for many years): 'Physical activity is crucially important for improving overall health and fitness levels. But there is limited evidence to suggest that it can blunt the surge in obesity'.[69]

---

68 Williams and Wood, 2006.
69 Loyola University Health System, 2015.

This is just another example of how primitive calories in/calories out reasoning does not take into account the impact of food and exercise on your metabolism and your hormones. Particularly if you are overweight or obese, go very gently with exercise in the early stages of your new dietary approach. Katy bought a simple pedometer so that she could control the number of steps she walked. Parking a bit further away when at the supermarket or gently riding a bicycle for short distances just kept her a little more active – nothing strenuous, however!

Health Booster 2:
Respect your biological time clock

Before artificial lighting existed, the sun was our major light source, so evenings were spent in the relative darkness of candlelight. We woke with the sun and slept with the stars, meaning that we probably got more sleep in the winter months.

With the recent advances made with LED lightbulbs, access to cheaper and brighter lighting is spreading. It will soon be available to all humanity – yet we may be paying a price for all that light. The body's biological clock, our so-called circadian rhythm, is confused and disturbed by so much evening light. As a result, sleep suffers. Recent evidence even suggests possible links to heart disease, cancer, diabetes and obesity.[70] In 1981, Dr Charles Czeisler of the Harvard Medical School showed that daylight keeps a person's internal clock aligned with their environment.[71] You can reduce your stress levels, it seems, simply by showing more respect for your natural circadian rhythm.

It is primarily the blue wavelengths, which aid our ability to pay attention during daylight, that seem to be most disruptive at night. Yet with TVs, tablets, smartphones and energy-efficient lighting all increasing our exposure to blue wavelengths, things are getting worse. Exposure to light suppresses the secretion of melatonin, a hormone that influences our circadian rhythm, and there's some experimental evidence showing that lower melatonin levels are associated with cancer. But research studies, including a 2011 Harvard study,[72] have also established a very real connection to diabetes and obesity. Ten people were put on a daily schedule that gradually shifted the timing of their circadian rhythms, leaving them with higher blood sugar levels and reduced levels of leptin – the hormone that helps register fullness.

---

70   Dodson and Zee, 2010.
71   Czeisler, 2006.
72   Harvard T.H. Chan School of Public Health, 2015.

Before we go to sleep, as well as toning down the light, our bodies and digestive systems need to wind down. So, two hours before that time, you need to have stopped eating and drinking anything caffeine-rich or alcoholic and have abstained from looking at TVs and other electronic screens. If you are comfortably getting your seven to eight hours of restful sleep, that's fine – but if not, follow these wind-down rules and read a good book before bed – preferably one printed on paper!

Your Circadian Sleep Tips:

Use dim red lights for night lights.

Avoid looking at bright screens, beginning two to three hours before bed.

Download a computer programme such as f.lux,[73] which adjusts your screen colour to warmer tones if you do need to use it in the evening.

Get exposed to bright light during the day – it will boost both your ability to sleep at night and your mood and alertness during the day.

---

73 www.justgetflux.com

Health Booster 3:
Stay hydrated ... by also eating your veggies

You'll often find the statement that drinking eight glasses of water a day is good for your diet and for your general health. In fact, a quick trawl of the internet will show you that this feat can also make you look sexier and younger, and can act as a body-detox to make you feel more energised. But Aaron E Carroll, Professor of Pediatrics and Assistant Dean for Research Mentoring at Indiana University School of Medicine, is one of a growing number who question its importance. He says that when originally coming up with this recommendation, scientists included the amount of fluid that you get through other food and vegetables. They never intended for people to drink eight glasses of water on top of their daily food and drink. 'There is no science behind it,' he wrote recently in the *New York Times*.[74]

On the other hand, drinking around a pint of water (just over half a litre) before each meal can help obese people lose weight, say researchers at the University of Birmingham in England[75] ... presumably because you then eat less! The researchers monitored eighty-four obese people for twelve weeks and found that those who 'pre-loaded' water before all three main meals lost an average of 4.3kg. Those who only 'pre-loaded' once, or not at all, lost an average of just 0.8kg.

The 'drink eight glasses' myth seems to originate in a 1945 US Food and Nutrition Board recommendation that people need about 2.5 litres of water a day.[76] Even though the next sentence read: 'Most of this quantity is contained in prepared foods', this part seems to have been glossed over.

Water makes up about 60% of your body weight, so no-one disputes that hydration is important. This is where another role comes in for

---

74   Carroll, 2015.
75   Parretti et al., 2015.
76   Valtin, 2002.

vegetables. Vegetables contain lots of water, with cucumber and lettuce topping the list at a remarkable 96% water. Courgettes, radish and celery follow with 95%; tomatoes with 94%; and even those denser-looking vegetables such as cauliflower, broccoli, eggplant, red cabbage and peppers consist of more than 90% water.

If you do work out gently and are considering one of those sugary sports drinks, it's good to know that you re-hydrate more quickly when munching on some cucumber or watermelon (92% water). When interviewed by the *Daily Mail* in 2009, Dr Susan Shirreffs of Loughborough University said:[77] 'To be properly hydrated, you need to replace fluid lost from the body with one that's similar to the body's natural composition. Watery fruit & vegetables often contain levels of minerals and sugar that mirror this, so they can hydrate you more effectively than water alone'. One thing is clear: you really don't need the sugary excess of a sports drink to help you.

In the big scheme of things, perhaps your best bet is to simply make sure you are well-hydrated by munching on vegetables and drinking water from time to time. But if you want to lose weight, maybe the time at which you drink your water is more important than how much you drink. As for Katy, her preferred snack was to munch on some cucumber – but depending on availability, you might also consider watermelon; it also brings with it the benefits of being one of those fruits with the lowest sugar content.

---

77   Stephens, 2009.

Attention: Carb warning …
from the *fatisourfriend.com* blog, March 2014[78]

Be careful in selecting your low-carb British breakfast:

Yesterday, I went to my local cafe and ordered a full English breakfast. It was an eye-opener. What should have been the perfect low-carb start to the day was in fact a high-carb bombshell. The price – £7.50 – was not cheap at all. The contents?

Well … on the healthier side, there was one poached egg (organic, they said), two sausages, half a grilled tomato and two rashers of bacon. Somewhere in the middle of the carb spectrum, there was a generous portion of baked beans. On the high-carb side, there was a large portion of bubble & squeak (fried mashed potato with a little low-carb cabbage, for those not in the know), one piece of fried bread, and, next to it, two pieces of buttered toast with a plastic covered mini-portion of marmalade.

Bearing in mind that the carb content of the sausages was probably over 10% and the beans were on the sweeter side, this was not a good start to the day. Just for the record, I skipped the toast and the fried bread but tried some of the 'bubble'. I have to admit, it was delicious – lots of butter, I suspect, and maybe about 20% cabbage – so slightly lower-carb than first impressions!

Here are some guidelines if you want to construct your own low-carb English breakfast:

- Two slices bacon (50g): 4g fat, 11g protein, no carbs.

- One *Wall's* brand sausage (50g): 9g fat, 6g protein, 6g carbs (lower in carbs if it's an all-meat sausage, of course; it's lowest if you target 90% plus).

- One large fried egg (50g): 7g fat, 6g protein, no carbs.

---

78   http://www.fatisourfriend.com/blog/full-english-can-be-problematic

- One portion mushrooms (100g): 1g fat, 4g protein, 4g carbs.

- One portion fried tomato (100g): 1g fat, 1g protein, 4g carbs.

Be careful with the following:

- Baked beans (small 50g portion): 2g fat, 3g protein, 7g carbs.

- Bread (1 slice): 1g fat, 3g protein, 13g carbs.

- Fried potatoes (hash browns) (100g): 13g fat, 3g protein, 32g carbs (bubble and squeak – a bit less).

My summary: you can make it 'oh so low-carb and healthy', but you'll certainly have to skip the bread and potatoes.

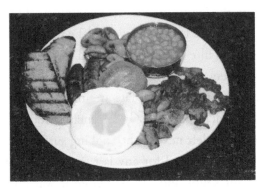

Figure 5:   Looks good …
but toast, fried potatoes, beans and carb-rich sausages are to be avoided.

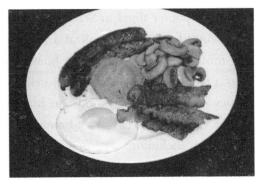

Figure 6 :   Still a fine, filling breakfast; just make sure the sausages are at least 90% meat to ensure a delicious low-carb start to the day.

Home economies

One criticism of low-carb, high-fat diets is that they are said to cost more – at least when you are purchasing food. As in most rumours of this kind, there is some truth in it – but not a lot.

By taking more food preparation into your own hands, you can save money if you're both clever with your purchases and if you heed the advice your grandparents or great-grandparents would have given. Let's take the Sunday roast. In those days when meat was both more expensive and scarcer, only the very rich would eat meat more than once or twice a week. The Sunday roast meal of beef, pork, lamb or occasionally chicken was served first to the family, before the remaining cold meat was sliced up to provide sustenance for the next day. The residual fat or 'dripping' that was left over was filtered and then added to whatever other residual fat was maybe still remaining from the previous week. It didn't even need to be kept cool since such animal fats are inherently stable and have a long shelf life. Animal fats don't easily go rancid at room temperature, so this fat could easily be left next to the cooking surface for everyday use. The carcass was then plucked for any last small pieces of meat (which would be saved for soups and salads) before it was boiled with some aromatic vegetable such as onion or celery to form a stock (bone-broth).

This was used as the base for the soup or portion-wise for sauces during the next days. In poorer times in Scotland, it was even done to pass on the boiled bones for a second boil at a neighbour's house. If you want to know more, it's worth reading the book *Nourishing Broth, written* by Dr Kaayla Daniel with Sally Fallon Morell and published in 2014.[79] Good recipes and lots of explanations! Such advocates of bone-broths claim that the valuable nutrients in a home-made stock lead to numerous health benefits, including:

---

79   Morell and Daniel, 2014.

1. Less joint pain.

2. Anti-inflammatory effect all over the body.

3. A reduction in infection caused by colds and flu viruses (chicken soup has been known for centuries as 'Jewish penicillin').

4. Helps bones grow stronger and healthier – the collagen allows for a greater absorption of minerals such as calcium.

5. Good for your hair and nails because of the natural gelatine in the broth.

How low can you go?
Going ketogenic for quicker weight loss

Dropping your intake of carbohydrates is one thing, but what happens when you go really low, dropping that level to below 20 grams per day? For a day or so, the body will use up its glycogen reserves, stored in your liver, before accessing proteins in the form of muscles or your fat reserves to produce the energy it needs. To keep going, your clever liver then begins to manufacture ketones for its basic fuel – an entirely normal process which was much-needed by our ancient forebears when meals were less frequently available than they typically are today.

This carbohydrate restriction begins the shift in your body's metabolism away from glucose towards fat utilisation. When eating a high-carb diet, your body chooses glucose for its fuel. But, with a restricted intake, you begin to use fat for fuel and go into what is technically called ketosis. Your insulin levels self-regulate at a lower level, your body accesses body fat for fuel and generally speaking you will experience weight-loss! As with all lower-carb diet methods, the better control of your blood sugar levels also leads to fewer pangs of hunger and sweet cravings.

Complete fasting (just water and no food at all) will also induce this process whereby your brain, for example, is no longer fuelled by glucose but by ketones. Yet, when it comes to losing weight, most of us don't have the will-power or the social environment which allow the rigours of fasting to represent a good choice.

That being said, as an accessible form of fasting, the medical theory behind ketosis is not new. The Ancient Greeks knew that fasting was a useful treatment for helping people cope with epileptic seizures. A little more recently, at one of the annual meetings of the American Medical Association, an endocrinologist named Dr Henry Rawle Geyelin first delivered a talk on therapeutic fasting and its connection with the treatment of epileptic seizures.[80] That was the summer of 1921. Now, getting on for a hundred years later, he might be surprised to find that the same basic dietary approach is used more often than not in connection with weight loss. In 1997, the film director Jim Abrahams made a film, First Do No Harm, starring Meryl Streep. It was based on his son's successful experiences with this ketogenic approach. Epilepsy and other diseases connected with inflammation in the body are certainly helped by an overall reduction in food intake – but it is the reduction of carbohydrates and upping of fat levels in the diet which do the trick. Patients like Jim Abraham's son Charlie can continue to eat well, but (as you will know by now) cream, cheese, butter, meats, fish, nuts and leafy vegetables replace the pasta, bread and sugar.

Dr Courtney Craig, who suffered with chronic fatigue syndrome for many years, refers to this dietary approach as a kind of spring-clean for the body, with old cells and decomposed tissue being burned away in the process. She advocates its use in connection with a number of medical conditions.[81] Your body gets rid of toxins and metabolic waste while producing ketones for your necessary brainpower (rather than glucose) as it begins to target your fat reserves. In a way, you are cannibalising your fat reserves. This approach has been made popular more recently, since it provides the basis for the initial phase of the Atkins diet. The process of burning fat is referred to as lipolysis. This, in turn, leads to ketosis – namely that low-carb state where your liver begins to produce ketones.

But this approach is not just about 'self-cannibalisation', because the body also goes into repair mode. Some researchers believe that ketosis even reboots the immune system.[82] Doing the high-carb opposite, for example, by adding just a tiny amount of glucose to worms' diets, has been found to shorten their lifespan by 20%.[83] Mice lead longer lives when carbs in their diet are reduced dramatically[84] – so could ketosis help

---

80   See Wheless, 2004, p.33.
81   Craig, 2015.
82   Paddock, 2014.
83   Lee, 2009.
84   Mattson, 2005.

us humans too? Soviet doctors showed in the 1950s that fasting could successfully treat asthma, and Western doctors nowadays are more likely to induce ketosis to cure epilepsy and improve disorders such as multiple personality syndrome. If you are interested, there is an informative short video available on YouTube called *The Science of Fasting*.[85]

Might the real problem here be that reducing carb intake or even fasting for a few days does not cost money and brings little profit to others? Some would say you need to be medically supervised if you take the more strict, ketogenic approach. But let's face it, thousands of people have followed this as the initial Atkins dietary stage with success. While it's always best to work in cooperation with your medical adviser, he or she is unlikely to be the one advising you to go ketogenic. The simple fact is that there's no money in promoting an approach like this for Big Pharma. Dr Andreas Michalsen from Europe's largest public hospital, the Charité hospital in Berlin, has written extensively on the subject of moderate fasting – the process they use to stimulate the ketogenic situation in which your body synthesises ketones to provide energy as opposed to converting carbs into glucose. They have forty-four beds at their Integrative Medicine and Naturotherapy department, which he heads up, and it is there that they regularly apply methods of fasting to treat complaints ranging from rheumatic arthritis to high blood pressure. One thing is quite clear when fasting: levels of leptin (the fullness sensitivity hormone) go up, while insulin goes down. When talking of his results, he says:[86] 'If I had been studying a new drug and got these results, I would be getting phone calls every day. It is very easy for critics to say there are not enough studies when we know there is no funding for these studies'. But there again, who would fund his research?

However, these low-carb and fasting approaches are becoming more mainstream. At Johns Hopkins University, they have run The Ketogenic Diet Center for many years. Their high-fat, low-carbohydrate ketogenic regime has been managed through the Paediatric Epilepsy team at Johns Hopkins since Dr Geyelin's time in the 1920s. Over the years, they have

---

85   Viadecouvertesprod, 2011.
86   Speaking in *The Science of Fasting* documentary.

enrolled hundreds of children on the ketogenic diet as well as a modified version of the Atkins diet. Patients ranging from infants to adolescents are admitted for a four-day period during which the diet is started and education provided. They have a particular focus on using their modified Atkins diet for epilepsy in clinical trials, but also have a diet wing for both children and adults and refer to themselves as the premier centre in the world for clinical and research expertise regarding the ketogenic diet.

Is it safe to go ketogenic?

If you decide to try this more aggressive cut-back in carbs, it is best to inform your doctor, although you can manage it yourself should you choose to. That's what Katy did, and apart from the self-discipline needed for the first few days and the occasional headache it suited her well. Some people report feeling nauseated and even exhibiting flu-like symptoms for a couple of days. This may be the result of electrolytes being flushed out of your body together with excess water, so having some good old chicken broth handy can be useful.

Katy restricted her diet to the 'Ketogenic Yes List' and, most importantly, did not feel hungry while eating this way. She did not specifically count her carbs, but we estimated that she was running at between 15 and 30 grams per day when we reviewed what she was eating. Two weeks into this more extreme form of low-carbing, she reported above all increased energy levels – more 'get up and go', she would say. Yet after a few weeks, to be frank, she got a bit bored. That's when some of the 'good for you' foods were added, particularly berries in small quantities. After all, as a Belgian, she had been used to delicious foods and sauces developed for taste rather than the primary thought process being about the ingredients. The high-fat principle worked for her, though, as did low-carb. What she initially missed was sweet pastries and cakes, but the occasional piece of dark chocolate helped her through.

If you're going ahead with a more dramatic weight loss approach like Katy did, it can be done safely as long as you keep to a broad base of items you select from the 'permitted' list, which is either no-carb or very low-carb.

The stricter 'Ketogenic No List' includes:

- All fruit, potatoes, breads, rice and most processed foods.

- Beans and legumes (including chickpeas).

- Milk, regular yoghurt, ice cream and cottage cheese. Check your 100% almond milk or soy milk because of the probable sugar content.

- All 'energy' or 'nutrition' bars.

- All beer and most alcohol, except the driest wines and spirits such as vodka or whisky (in limited quantities because although they contain very few carbs, your body will seek out the alcohol as an energy source before using protein and fat. Avoiding them will also take the burden off your liver).

- Fizzy drinks/soda – including diet drinks.

- Honey, maple syrup, artificial sweeteners and stevia (only as exceptions).

- Processed meats unless artisanal.

The 'Ketogenic Yes List' includes:

- Eggs – so many different ways; Katy's favourite was hard-boiled mimosa eggs in salads, with differing mayo-based fillings.

- Cheese (real cheese – not processed types such as cheese slices). The best are aged harder cheeses.

- Other dairy including heavy cream, sour cream, butter; full-fat Greek yoghurt in smaller quantities.

- Olives – choose black ones for lowest carb levels.

- All meats are fine unless cured in sugar/honey. Salted meats are fine; go for the best bacon you can afford and 100% meat sausages – they're best from your butcher.

- All vegetables except sweetcorn, potatoes and other root vegetables.

- Sauerkraut and other fermented foods; pickled onions and gherkins.

- Fish and shellfish – but if you eat sushi, set the rice aside.

- Pure vegetable juice, including tomato and carrot – but limit the quantities. They have some carbs but the benefits exceed the downside!

- All nuts and seeds – including peanut butter and coconut (limited quantities).

- All oils, vinegar, home-made mayonnaise and mustard – but no ketchup.

- Spices and herbs; lemon and lime in small quantities.

- Stay well-hydrated by drinking water and herbal teas/tisanes. Coffee is OK (a dash of cream in your coffee is fine, but no milk).

Useful tips

A ketogenic diet is still considered extreme by many doctors, although in real life, there are few (if any) reported cases of people who have suffered any severe consequences. It's best to check you have no unusual underlying conditions before you start, though diabetes indicators may of course be what you're trying to improve. A keto-diet can take many forms, but if you count the carbs, it usually involves restricting carbohydrates to less than 50 g per day. A useful guide to a ketogenic diet is to follow the 60/35/5 rule where 60% of calories come from fat, 35% from protein, and just 5% from carbs. That compares with a typical Western diet, which these days is about 15% protein, 15 to 25 % fat, and anything between 60 and 70% carbohydrates.

That being said, what do you do if your doctor doesn't approve of a very low-carb ketogenic diet? It's best to ask your doctor what evidence he/she would need to change their mind. If your doctor says that their mind cannot be changed, that's problematic. You might have to consider finding a new doctor. A sensible and more rational answer might lead to a blood or urine test, which will almost certainly work out in your favour. While you are on your more extreme version of the diet, you can still run into social problems. Here are some of Katy's tips, based on problems she experienced:

Problem: Carbs, particularly sweet ones, can look really appetizing – True, but if you are hungry, make yourself a meal from the approved list and you will quickly lose your appetite for the carbs.

Problem: You may have eaten carbs in differing forms, from corn flakes to chocolate bars, as ways to wind down or de-stress over the years – If you feel depressed or anxious, find a quiet place to sit or lie down where you can let yourself feel all of your emotions. If you still want some comfort food, try just two pieces of dark (85%) chocolate or eat some salted nuts.

Kathryn's Salad Niçoise

A beautiful low-carb summer salad with pine nuts replacing the boiled potatoes ~ don't worry; you won't miss them.

Ingredients (for four people):
- 4 large eggs.
- 200g fine green beans.
- 200g baby tomatoes.
- 250g lettuce leaves.
- 100g sliced pitted black olives.
- 1 x 200g can of tuna (natural or in olive oil, but avoid sunflower oil).
- 4 tbs extra-virgin olive oil.
- Juice of half a lemon.
- Salt and pepper to taste.
- 30g pine nuts.
- 4 anchovy fillets.
- 30g fresh basil leaves.

Method:
1. Put the eggs in a saucepan of cold water and bring to a boil for 4 minutes. During this time, add the beans.
2. Remove the beans and place in cold water to keep them 'al-dente' while letting the eggs cool naturally in the water.
3. Chop the baby tomatoes in half. Mix briskly with the olives in the oil, lemon juice, salt and pepper.
4. Arrange the chopped lettuce on a serving dish. Top with the tomato-olive mixture and add chunks of the strained tuna and beans.
5. Peel and quarter the hard-boiled eggs and add them. Add the anchovy fillets and basil leaves before sprinkling with pine nuts.

Problem: You're out in public and feel pressured to join in with the cake or ice cream (at my school, this was a recurrent theme with all the birthdays!) – Try a variation on a white lie; one that may well be anchored in the truth. Say that your doctor has told you that you're developing insulin resistance, so you cannot eat sugary foods for a while. No one will try and countermand your doctor's instructions.

Problem: You're at an event that only serves carb-rich food such as sandwiches and pizza – What's best is to eat before the event so you're not actually hungry, otherwise you'll have to pretend to be full. But don't fall into the trap of saying: 'Oh I'd love to eat one but …', because someone will surely succeed in tempting you!

Katy's success factors for those first ten days

Whatever you do, don't go hungry. In fact, after a while on this diet, you won't feel hungry. Don't worry about your fat intake or cholesterol levels, forget the low-fat bandwagon and don't even think of counting calories.

Be disciplined – you can do it!

Go shopping before you start, and remove all temptation from your fridge and cupboards. Plan on eating as much as possible at home, and prepare packed lunches as needed (salad jars are a favourite).

Prepare some snack foods in case you have the desire to eat; I used celery sticks dipped in cream cheese and also individual chicory leaves with a little Roquefort cream and half a walnut – but that's just me! After a few days, I stopped snacking anyway.

Organic bouillon cubes came in handy too, for hot drinks.

Drink lots of water and avoid too much exercise. Gentle walking was enough.

Write down how you feel on day one and then write down your energy level on day ten – you'll see the difference! How about sleep quality and your mood?

Measure your waist and hips (that's halfway between your hipbone and your lowest rib) after five days and after ten days. Weigh yourself at the same intervals – but not every day!

After day ten:

You can start adding small amounts of carbohydrates back into your diet – such as small pieces of fresh fruit, some cooked lentils or a few more nuts.

Continue to stay away from all refined sugars and white flours! 'Working at a school meant that learning to say "No" at the frequent birthday celebrations was difficult for me, but I did it,' says Katy.

As you add in more carbs, you may find that bloating returns. You may feel a bit depressed or even experience short-term lower energy levels. This is natural as your body establishes its new set-point or balance level for the proportions of carbs you can eat while staying happy, motivated and leaner.

Unpleasant side effects? Yes; in the early stage, you may experience bad breath if your body switches right over from burning carbs to 'cannibalising' its own fat from your body – but that will pass. Maybe you'll experience a rumbling tummy, but your overall digestion should soon benefit from this way of eating. You may feel irritable, even lethargic, before your energy levels increase. But again, that will pass. And those energy levels will increase.

The more your body is used to getting its quick-burning energy from sugar and refined flour the more likely you are to also experience headaches as you kick your sugar habit – but it's worth it. Katy summarises it this way: 'The benefits included weight loss and increased energy for me but improved sleep quality and reduced joint pain were, I think, also associated with the results'.

A word on 'FODMAPs'

One extra note – about avoiding FODMAPs. It's a strange word for a very select group of carbohydrates that just may be poorly absorbed by your small intestine. If you suffer from food allergies and symptoms such as a bloated stomach and indigestion but still have a clear desire to lose weight, it's a word you best get familiar with – and it might mean starting your diet with a stricter approach. There's lots of information online these days about FODMAPs; they are listed as foods you need to avoid because they are potentially adding to your digestive problems. Many people find that cutting out carbs, processed foods and gluten is enough to generate big improvements, but avoiding FODMAPs is an approach from which many have benefited. If you decide to be more restrictive in your dietary options, you can still learn from Katy's diet. After a few weeks, you can begin to slowly add in some of the foods you have eliminated – but skipping all wheat-based breads may be something you have to live with long-term. If you get used to a low-carb, high-fat lifestyle, you won't miss them much in any case!

The FODMAPs acronym refers to Fermentable Oligo-saccharides, Disaccharides, Monosaccharides and Polyols. What a mouthful! These are the tiny molecules found in food that can be mal-absorbed in the small intestine of your digestive tract before arriving at the large intestine, where they act as nourishment for the bacteria that live there. For some people, this causes a number of unpleasant symptoms, from bloating to IBS to even skin rashes.

This may be too much information for you, but the small bowel, which connects the stomach to the large bowel, is around six metres long. Relatively few bacteria normally live there, and the bacteria which are present are also different from those present in the colon. When doing its job correctly, the small bowel plays an important role in digesting food and helps you absorb nutrients. It also benefits your immune system. Although bacteria are an essential part of a healthy small bowel and perform important functions, small intestinal bacterial overgrowth can lead to leaky gut and potentially to other symptoms.

Since bacteria eat the starch contained in cereals and grains, this provides a possible explanation why avoiding all grains, not just those with gluten, helps many people – even when they are not truly 'allergic' to gluten. The funny (or not so funny) thing is, many gluten-free products contain flour from beans and legumes, which are not allowed according to the FODMAPs list – so they may be irritating you.

FODMAPs, especially free fructose, are thought to promote rapid fermentation and lead to potential abdominal bloating. Incidentally, each of us absorbs and digests fructose a bit differently. This is why, to this day, I limit the amount of fresh fruit that I eat.

This more restricted list of foods is supported by many who advocate a paleo-style diet, which features foods that people ate before the birth of agriculture ten to twelve thousand years ago. Arguably, the diet we evolved to eat over millions of years consisted of meat, fish, eggs, vegetables, nuts and low-sugar fruits such as berries. In moderate climates, fruits like fructose-rich bananas or mangoes simply did not exist; our switch to a diet heavy in grains (which are essentially grasses) in the form of pasta and breads is relatively recent. Many of you may be aware of such paleo diet approaches, which are sometimes also known under the term 'caveman diet'. It was, after all, Google's most searched-for weight loss method in 2013. Advocates also argue against the use of added sugars and chemical additives, which dates back only a couple of hundred years at most. Paleo diet advocates suggest that this has led to a huge increase in auto-immune health problems ranging from bowel disorders to obesity, diabetes and cancer.[87] Their many websites can provide a useful resource.

As such, a FODMAPs-free diet may be a necessary step back before embarking again on a more varied diet. I would suggest and recommend that the grains and added sugars associated with mass-produced food today are kept to a minimum for the long-term. Get further information from your doctor, or read the brief Stanford University guide.[88] I can also

---

87   Connor, 2014.
88   Stanford Hospital and Clinics, 2015.

recommend visiting the website of Natasha Campbell-McBride at www. gapsdiet.com.

PART 4

THE REAL ROSETO EFFECT

Another time, another place

About the same time that I was 'consulting' Katy, a long-weekend break took me to that lesser-known part of Italy, in their deep South, Puglia – or as it's more commonly known in English, Apulia.

Living where I do, just south of Brussels in the old battle town of Waterloo (please don't start humming that Abba song), we are within easy reach of Charleroi airport – or what the marketing people at Ryanair charmingly refer to as 'Brussels South'. With access to cheap flights heading towards sunnier parts of Europe, my wife and I selected a short break in Southern Italy, landing in Bari, the local capital city. Puglia is the large, fertile and heavily agricultural region that forms the heel of Italy's boot, being quite flat and surrounded by sea in the South and yet with mountainous terrain in the North West. Proximity to clean beaches, guaranteed sunshine and a distinct lack of non-Italian tourists seemed to make it a worthy destination, but for me there was an added attraction – food! Not just pizza and pasta, but menus featuring a strong local influence, supported in part by government measures.

With many people leaving their small-scale farm houses for the cities in the 1950s, '60s and '70s, the Italian government seized the initiative to pass a law that defined something called *agriturismus*. This law allowed small farmers to supplement their farm's income with the provision of accommodation for tourists and the offer of food and drink – all (at least to some extent) tax-advantaged. As a result, during the last thirty to forty years, many previously abandoned buildings and estates have been restored – some to luxurious levels, with hotel-style service and even infinity swimming pools. One thing you can be sure of finding in all these establishments, regardless of price, is excellent freshly made food – most of it sourced from local ingredients on the farms.

It was while doing a little pre-travel research and looking for some fine *agriturismo* destinations that I came across a village name that I recognised, Roseto. At first I couldn't place it, but then I remembered that the Roseto I had heard of was in rural Pennsylvania in the United States. The author and social commentator, Malcolm Gladwell, had written about the unique healthy aspects of that small American town in the middle part of the twentieth century in his book, *Outliers: The Story of Success*, which was a big publishing hit in 2008.[89] The book was on my shelf, so I took the opportunity to refresh my memory – rediscovering that Roseto was the very first all-Italian township established in the United States, and that the early inhabitants had all emigrated from that very same village of Roseto in the foothills behind Bari, Puglia.

A visit to Puglia stimulates all the visual senses – and it also stimulates the taste buds. The cooking, aligned with the fresh local ingredients, is simple and unpretentious – and not exactly what you'd describe as low-carb. Locally grown semolina flour is made into many different handmade pastas, the most famous being Orecchiette (shaped like little ears), which is served up together with local greens and pureed fava beans or tossed with a hearty meat ragout. A wide variety of wild and cultivated greens are used, ranging from sorrel to broccoli raab and dandelions, lengthy cooking being needed to soften them. Rustic breads – mostly leavened but some unleavened – are baked daily. Many dishes, whether appetizers, mains or salads, are doused (at least these days) in olive oil; Puglia being Italy's largest olive oil producer. I say 'these days' simply because, historically, olive oil was used primarily as a source of fuel and lighting – the huge and numerous underground olive presses on exhibit in Gallipoli paying testament to that today. When it came to food, at most, olive oil was used as a salad dressing.

With a long history of shepherding animals in the North, the Apulians, as they are known, cook with lamb and goat meat. They eat the whole animal, with even lambs' hearts being skewered and cooked on a grill – a particular local favourite. They like to eat this together with raw celery and sharp sheep's milk cheese. Greens as a separate dish or on a side plate can be served as a puree of fava beans, folded into pasta or dropped into soups. They love their fava beans, which are widely used and served in many different ways.

---

89   Gladwell, 2008.

More fish is eaten the closer to the coast you get. In the ports of Taranto and Gallipoli in the South, sea urchins are eaten raw, flavoured with just a squeeze of lemon to balance their briny taste. Desserts reflect the region's rich cultural heritage (a history of trading combined with multiple invasions), Puglia having been a major stopping point for travellers over the centuries – particularly those from Greece and further east. Honey, nuts and dried fruit are key ingredients in pastries, cakes and fried desserts, giving an oriental touch to the end of a meal.

While planning my vacation, I also found out that the very first Gothic novel ever written was based there. Horace Walpole's *The Castle of Otranto* was written way back in the early 1760s. It tells the fictional story of Manfred of Sicily's son being crushed to death on his wedding day by a gigantic helmet ... and all that ensues. Although Horace Walpole got as far as Naples on his own grand tour of Italy, there is no record of him ever visiting Otranto. Indeed, at that time, with no railway transport across the hills, going south from Naples to Taranto and on to Otranto and Lecce would have been very time-consuming. Otranto is almost as far south as you can get in South Eastern Italy, and (as I would later discover) a visit to the real castle provides beautiful scenic views across the Adriatic to Albania on a clear day. When I visited, the castle's summer exhibition showed many paintings resulting from those *grand tours taken by* the aristocracy and other young, well-to-do European men of means in the eighteenth and nineteenth centuries. It was seen as an educational rite of passage; a kind of finishing school in art and manners.

The collection of hundreds of pictures shows mainly local people eating, drinking and enjoying themselves in social situations. We must consider them to be an idealised insight into real life in the sense that Puglia, with no main river for irrigation and highly dependent on trade, was a poor and far-flung area of the country. While observing those pictures which showed cooking and eating, I identified many fresh fruit and vegetables as well as goats and lambs and even pigs. But, hard as I looked, there was no visual reference to the use of olive oil – except, that is, in the context of lamps for use in the evenings ... which takes me back to the town of Roseto.

It's funny how the mind makes connections – I remembered reading that even in the 1950s and '60s, the Rosetans (who had originally sought out a better life in Pennysylvania) were described as being unable to afford olive oil like their forebears in Italy, having to use lard in their pastries and for frying. 'In spite of that', said the doctors writing about their unhealthy diet (they categorised it as 'rich in cholesterol and animal fat'[90]), those Italian descendants lived longer lives freer from heart disease when compared to their American counterparts living just a few miles away. Yet the more I looked into it, the more I found that cooking with olive oil is a twentieth and twenty-first century phenomenon. True, in the past, the rich had access to olive oil and used it on some salads (as maybe did poorer people for special occasions), but olive oil was fundamentally needed for lighting and heating and sometimes for medicinal and cosmetic purposes.

Today, olive oil is touted by nutrition experts around the world as the very cornerstone of the healthy Mediterranean diet. But (although I do not dispute that it represents a good oil to cook with) go back a few generations and this simply wasn't the case because it was needed for other purposes. Gallipoli, in the south of Puglia, was the world's centre for the olive oil trade between the seventeenth and nineteenth centuries. But what they sold was named, best-quality lamp-oil – and it was quoted as such on the British stock market in London until the 1850s, when petrol and electricity were in their infancy. Don't go thinking these were the cheap left-overs they were selling, either. The major trade was in high-quality virgin olive oil, primarily because it gave off less smoke when burned.

My first encounter in the UK with olive oil consisted of a doctor warming it and putting some in my ear to help relieve an earache. But why is all this of any relevance? Because those residents of Roseto in the USA were apparently some of the healthiest Americans that have ever lived. The question is: was this in spite of their diet? Or perhaps (at least in part) *because* of their diet? I wanted to find out, and you can read the full story in Part 8. But suffice it to say that just as I was reading up on

---

90   Moss, 2011, p.218.

the healthy benefits of eating more freshly prepared food and lowering your carb intake, my study of the folks in Roseto showed me that healthy saturated fats were also a part of the mix. My experience of the local cookery in the Italian town of Roseto and its surroundings today – where lard is still used in pastry and eating offal is quite normal – support this thinking. When originally reviewed by doctors and sociologists in the 1960s, the secret of the Rosetans' heart-friendly existence was put down entirely to that tightly knit social infrastructure inherited from the Italian ethos they had brought with them from the original Roseto. Since the 1960s, they have slowly but steadily rejoined regular American society. As a largely commuter town, these days – health-wise – they are no different from their neighbours. The cohesion of their family social structure has broken down and their diet has become truly American – fast-food, high-carb, low-fat and all.

The eventual diet I prescribed for Katy was further influenced by my experiences in Puglia and by the historical backdrop outlined here. Above all, it was the freshness and the diversity of foods that left an impression; that and the quantity and number of different vegetables used to create both expected and unexpected taste experiences, from bitter to sweet. Let's not forget that the wine they drink, mostly red, is also hearty and full-bodied and comes from rare and unusual grapes – which just add more to the biodiversity of their diet. The three major red varieties, two of which are grown nowhere else and can only be found in Puglia, are *Nero di Troia*, *Negroamaro* and *Primitivo*. They are dark red wines with a pleasant sweet ripe initial taste, yet some have a slightly bitter finish from the tannin.

I can only assume that with this dietary variety their digestive systems get by without the need for the prebiotic and probiotic supplements that our society increasingly seems to need when presented with the increasingly common standard American diet or its British equivalent. Above all, my visits to Puglia presented me with very few obese people on the streets – except, that is, for tourists and a certain fattening trend that's observable, sadly, among the younger members of society. While attending a cooking school just outside Bari, the regional capital of

Puglia, I met one young man who had returned to southern Puglia after studying in Milan, having put on 10 kilos in the process. His mother confronted him with the line: 'Pizza or pasta? One of them has to go!'. He subsequently gave up pizza and bread and has lost those 10 kilos. His mother's home cooking has, of course, also helped. I had the opportunity to ask her whether she ever counted calories. After much laughter, she asked why you would ever need to do that.

This brings us nicely on to our next subject. Why count calories when the studies show that 95% of those who start on calorie-controlled diets end them in failure? Many of them report even being heavier six months after the diet was over. If, as Einstein is reputed to have said, the definition of insanity is trying the same thing over and over and still expecting a different result, why do we keep on doing it?

PART 5

WHY COUNTING CALORIES USUALLY ENDS IN FAILURE

Just diet and exercise; you'll soon lose weight ...really?

The old and established mantra of weight loss depending on 'calories in versus calories out' is just plain not true. Glancing at the subject quickly, it seems blindingly obvious that energy eaten must equal energy expended; it's all about energy balance, after all. Right? Wrong. As we will see upon closer examination, it is quite obviously wrong. This is important, at least to me, because I have come to believe that our obsession with counting calories is one of the most important factors contributing to this unhealthy environment that's making us ill and adding inches to our waistlines.

Although we all know that some people put on weight more easily than others, those who get fat are often judged by society with phrases like: 'well, they didn't try hard enough, did they?' or 'they clearly lack self-discipline'. Yes, people really like to get on their high horses about this. 'Dieting? It all comes down to two things: eating less and exercising more,' said my friend Susan just the other day. In broader discussion groups, I've had the first law of thermodynamics thrown at me countless times – that's the one relating to conservation of energy, which says that the form of energy may change but the total is always conserved. So physicists agree: calories in must equal calories out. Except it's not quite true.

Let's say that you want to lose a kilo of fat from your body. We will first begin our weight reduction task with some exercise. It's quite easy arithmetic, really. You could work off that kilo by climbing the stairs in a five-thousand-storey building, you could run at a good pace for just 200 kilometres or – I am reliably informed – you could spend one enthralling sixteen-hour day, without pauses, cleaning out animal stalls ... if you could manage it. No wonder farm workers have such appetites!

It is quite true that you would lose weight after your efforts; most of it in the form of fat and water. That carbon-heavy body tissue would be converted into carbon dioxide and water vapour, so you would effectively get rid of the fat by breathing it out of your body. Yes, weight loss via exercise is possible – but you'll have gathered by now that it is not necessarily the easiest way of going about it.

Here's another way to look at weight loss in terms of what you could do exercise-wise today, if you wanted. Just go at it very hard for three hours continuously (swimming, running or cycling hard, for example). That will present you with the opportunity of losing about 100 grams of body fat. Lighter exercise such as walking fast or gardening works out at about 10 grams of fat (roughly a teaspoon) per hour ... although I'm struggling to picture that!

Your body fat is very dense and represents (so say the physicists) a bit less than 8,000 calories of energy per kilo, which is incidentally roughly the same energy density you will find in the petrol you put in your car. But when you try to cut back, first a word of warning: even light exercise contributes to the loss of half a litre of water or more per hour, so standing on the scale after sport might give you a false sense of satisfaction. Not forgetting, of course, that many of us have a bite to eat or a so-called energy drink after 'all that exercise' and end up increasing our body weight in the process! But that's another story.

Let's fast-forward to tomorrow. You're back on the scales, after your body has self-adjusted for the missing water, and you see to your great disappointment that the weight is back! Except it isn't, of course: you really did lose 20 or 30 grams, but your scales won't even begin to register this until a few days have gone by (unless you drank that sports drink or ate that sandwich, in which case there probably will be no reduction – maybe even a little weight gain). After all, didn't your Mum sometimes tell you as a child to go outside and run around to work up an appetite for dinner? Sadly, that works for adults too – exercise makes you feel hungry.

You might think on this the next time you see Coca-Cola or McDonalds promoting the football World Cup and the Olympic

Games. It is very much in their interest to show that exercise is closely linked to weight loss. Unsurprisingly, Coca-Cola, the founding sponsor of the 'Exercise is Medicine' initiative, preaches that sugary sodas are not a bad thing so long as you enjoy an active lifestyle.

Don't get me wrong; exercise is good for you. But you should exercise first and foremost to stay healthy or get healthier and only as a distant second to impact your weight.

From exercise, back to food. Now, according to the 'calories in, calories out' mantra, the specifics of what you eat are unimportant; counting calories is what counts! So, if you assume all calories are equal, eating a kilo of cooked broccoli will do the same to your body as eating a small-sized Snickers bar. Here, I have to tell you: I think you are wrong. Although they both represent about 350 calories of energy, we are simply not machines or engines that run on coal, oil or whatever. Our fuel (the food we eat) is very varied, our bodies have many needs and the ways we deal with snacks and meals and go about processing them are also varied.

Our reference point, that first law of thermodynamics, is all to do with conservation: it says that although the form of energy may change, the total is always conserved. Well, this may work in a physics lab or when trying to improve the efficiency of an internal combustion engine – but we are complex living beings with our own internal ecosystems. There are any number of variables involved which affect the relative efficiency of our bodily system – many of which are out of our control. That is why people never seem to gain or lose weight precisely as calculated – or have you found otherwise? No diet gets the same weight loss across a group of people; proof enough that calories in is not equating to calories out, you might think.

Let me return for the last time to what physicists in the lab describe as a thermodynamic system. Such a system includes kinetic energy, potential energy, internal energy and flow energy, as well as heat and work processes. I know this all sounds a bit scientific, but we can equate this to the way our human bodies generate and use energy. Some of the food we eat gets converted to energy and used in voluntary or involuntary movement; some generates extra heat that we need in colder climates or during winter; some becomes involved with inflammatory and infectious processes; some with growth, tissue restoration and numerous metabolic processes; some is absorbed by our digestive systems and some excreted; some is stored as fat; some is converted in the liver to glucose; and so on – not forgetting, of course, the complex interaction between these many activities. Let's also not forget the complex role that regulatory hormones and enzymes play and basic differences in metabolism (efficiency) between us humans, of which we are all aware. Some eat a lot and stay slim; some don't. But much of this is out of our direct control.

That first law of thermodynamics is a bookkeeping law and tells us that the total energy attributed to work, heat and changes in chemical composition will be constant. The second law is the one that drives chemical and biological reactions – and many, many such activities are at work inside our bodies. Just bear in mind that – according to the European Food Information Council (EUFIC) – we stroll around with around 1 kilo or more of gut bacteria quietly getting on with things.[91] We also excrete our own weight in faecal bacteria every year – yuck! You could even argue that we are not entirely human, in the sense that there's a complex ecosystem deep within us that is home to an amazing diversity of life – with very little of it belonging to our species. Of the around one hundred trillion organisms that live in your gut, the microbes outnumber their human counterparts by about two thirds. Recent evidence also indicates that these gut bacteria have a large effect on the way we store fat, how we balance levels of glucose in the blood and also (importantly) how we respond to those hormones, such as leptin, which make us feel hungry or full.

How much you eat is, of course, important – but counting it up in calories kind of misses the point. Eating too much over time on a daily basis will definitely affect you negatively. Many will put on weight, and many will, over time, get ill. Diabetes and non-alcoholic fatty liver disease – that's where more than 10% of the liver is made up of fat – are on the rise, and they are not just limited to the obese or even the overweight among us (that's most of us, by the way). Up to 30% of Americans

---

91   EUFIC, 2001.

already live with non-alcoholic fatty liver disease (NAFLD), according to experts.[92] In less than a decade, NAFLD will likely become the number one cause of liver transplants in the country, with demand continuing to overwhelm the supply of available livers.

An excess of carbohydrate in our diets, mostly in the form of processed starch and sugar, is leading to this. Yet measuring what we eat simply in terms of calories shifts the focus away from the quality of what we eat to the quantity. That's a mistake – and even if such an approach did lead to weight loss, what's the point of that if it is not linked to greater health?

---

92   Goff, 2012.

How calorie reduction disturbs your body and your mind

If you do simply look at your energy needs in terms of quantity, a reasonable daily diet for a man is around 2,400 calories of food. For a woman, it's around 2,000 calories. That equates to the energy that a conventional 100-watt light bulb expends in an hour. Much of what we eat goes to simple functions such as maintaining our own body temperature – so when you enter a room, you also warm the air much in the same way that a light bulb does.

During World War Two, the American scientist Ancel Keys took charge of a team of thirty-six conscientious objectors who agreed to cut their diet by over 1,000 calories per day for twenty-four weeks in support of the war effort. The reduction in food intake was to be combined with gentle exercise such as taking walks regularly. Known as the Minnesota Starvation Experiment,[93] the goal was to reduce their weight by around 25% per individual; a reduction of just over a kilo per week. There was a genuine scientific reason for this somewhat macabre experiment; namely, it was linked to the poor diets experienced by many in Europe during those wartime conditions and the lessons that could be learned.

Cut your consumption by 600 calories per day and you will lose around 0.5 kilo of fat every week according to the diet experts trained in the world of calorie counting – many of whom consider that a reasonable goal. That cut itself would represent a form of semi-starvation, but a 1,000-calorie reduction is definitely pushing the boundaries – as they found out back in 1945. What they discovered was that this prolonged semi-starvation diet did not just promote weight loss but produced significant increases in depression, hysteria and hypochondria (none of which I believe are covered by the laws of thermodynamics). They also saw decreases in each subject's basal metabolic rate (the energy required by the body in a state of rest) which were reflected in lower

93   Keys, 1950.

body temperature, slower breathing and reduced heart rate. All the volunteers survived, but it took most of them years to recover. What this study clearly demonstrated at the time was that diet alone will have a significant impact on your basic body functions such as blood pressure, cholesterol levels, resting heart rate, etc. – areas which were previously considered relatively fixed.

This was an unpleasant experience for the volunteers. First, they were permanently hungry and became obsessed with food, even during the recovery stage. Second, the psychological impact on them and their families was immense. With many popular calorie reduction schemes advocating a drop per day of around 600 calories over a prolonged period of time, you have to wonder about the cumulative psychological effect on these everyday dieting 'volunteers' too. There is no evidence I am aware of that links the process of being on a calorie-controlled diet to being a happier person.

It's worth taking note of these words from the World Health Organization:[94] 'Health is a state of complete physical, mental and social wellbeing and not merely the absence of disease or infirmity'. To paraphrase: if you go on a 'healthy' diet, it should be able to contribute to your physical, mental and social wellbeing. When it comes to successful dieting, my experience now tells me that around one-third is determined by what you eat, one-third by how much you eat and another third roughly divided between exercise and your God-given genetics. In other words: if you don't get the diet part right, you are not in a good place to start work on your exercise programme (if you choose to do so).

You can argue, as do the traditionally trained dieticians, that the quantity of food you eat trumps everything. But the remarkable fact is that (as we will see) if you eat the right foods, you do not feel hungry; you take charge and you make the decision to eat less rather than someone else telling you what to do. Your hormonal balance is restored. This has to be good, because you are more likely to stick to something if your body is sending regular positive messages.

94   World Health Organization, 1948. The Definition has not been amended since.

And let's remember that although it is very popular these days to blame your genes, Tim Spector, Professor of Genetic Epidemiology at King's College London is on record as saying:[95] 'You can influence your genetic make-up; you are not merely a slave to destiny, so that's one excuse out the window!'.

Let me introduce you to a new but relevant buzzword: nutrigenomics. Short for nutritional genomics, it is the study of how foods affect our genes and how individual genetic differences can affect the way we respond to the nutrients in the foods we eat. It turns out that what you eat can change how your genes are expressed and in so doing determine health outcomes – providing support for the 'you are what you eat' advocates.

Researchers now believe that:

Certain foods help activate the expression of good genes, switching off the bad ones and letting your body function in an improved, healthier way.

Eating particular refined carbohydrates and other constituents of a 'junk food' diet influences harmful genes, switching off the good ones and leading to poor health.

So the genes that you are born with seem to give you certain parameters to work with, but you can make the best of them – if you eat well. Which would be all well and good – if only the experts could agree on what eating well really meant and what precisely constitutes a healthy, balanced diet!

---

95   In Spector, 2012, Chapter 1: *The Gene Myth.*

Obesity – it's all relative

Obesity is relative; in the land of the obese, who is to say that lightweights represent the desired state? True, if you take the occasional peek at the Daily Mail, you will notice that bikinis and skinny people in varying degrees of underwear capture more column inches than that photo space given to porkier people; unless you are what the doctors variously describe as 'grotesquely' or 'morbidly' obese, in which case you become a photographic object of interest at the other end of the scale. Slim, muscle-toned bodies still represent the desired representation of the body fantastic – as, in many ways, they have done over the centuries. Just take a look at Michaelangelo's David.

But also consider the situation in Colorado – thought of as one of America's healthiest states. You may be unaware that Colorado is the skinniest of all the increasingly fat American States. The Rocky Mountain state has a smaller number of obese residents than any other in the USA. Yet the relatively low rate of obesity that they report now would have made Colorado the fattest state back in 1995, according to the latest report from the Robert Wood Johnson Foundation.[96] That's how fast the American waistline is currently expanding – but a supermarket visit in rural England or middle Germany will show how Europe is sadly trying as hard as it can to catch up with its American forerunners.

It is probably worth noting that Colorado doesn't have much reason to be happy with these 'skinny' results. It turns out that Colorado only leads the pack because of its ability to attract the healthy older adults moving in to enjoy the famed outdoor lifestyle that the state's reputation evokes. When you turn to the younger folks, there is (rather disappointingly) a different story to tell, with Colorado's rate of growth in childhood obesity being one of the worst in the nation!

So how do we generally measure 'fatness' in the twenty-first century? According to the BMI measurement criteria, a score that exceeds 30

---

96   Robert Wood Johnson Foundation, 2015.

equals obesity. In that context, how is Colorado doing? It seems that 19.8% of adults are obese; a figure which is up from 10.7% in 1995. Yet Colorado is now the last American state left with an obesity figure below 20%. Twelve US states even have obesity rates above 30%, most of them being in the American South.[97] Sad as this in itself, and even acknowledging the problems and inconsistencies with the official BMI system, these high obesity rates can be directly correlated with poor health. This takes the form of diabetes, high blood pressure, heart disease and other chronic illnesses. So if you're reading this from the comfort of a European home base, let's not get too smug about things. We are well on the way, in Europe, to emulating Colorado.

---

97   All statistics from www.stateofobesity.org

Diet, exercise or larger portion sizes?

According to the 'calories in, calories out' way of thinking, obesity is simply a matter of eating too many calories. The types of foods you eat aren't particularly important. If the only way to lose weight is to eat less and to move more, then it comes down to a person's individual responsibility to keep calories balanced. Put differently: if you get fat, it's your fault. Here's another way of looking at it. One kilogram represents 7700 calories, which would mean that if you ate 550 calories less than you burn per day for one week, you would lose exactly 0.5 kilo.

According to the US Department of Agriculture (USDA), in 1970 the food supply provided on average 2,039 calories per person per day. Yet by 2010, this amount had increased by more than 20% to 2,534 calories.[98] So, according to the principles of calories in equalling calories out, those extra 448 calories per day would add nearly 50 pounds (23 kilos) to the average adult in any given year. Over those forty years, using the simple average of a 224 calories increase per year (and all other things such as exercise levels being equal), an average twenty-year-old American would have put on 1,000 pounds (450 kilos) by the time they reached sixty.

Most Americans would have exploded long ago if this were indeed the case. Even allowing for a greater calorie need to maintain body weight as you get fatter, the accompanying more sedentary lifestyle that would be forced upon you would balance things out.

Europe's obesity league:
UK: 24.9%
Ireland: 24.5%
Spain: 24.1%
Portugal: 21.6%
Germany: 21.3%
Belgium: 19.1%
Austria: 18.3%
Italy: 17.2%
Sweden: 16.6%
France: 15.6%

Figure 7: From Measuring Up – a 2013 report on the UK's obesity crisis.

98   USDA Economic Research Service, 2015.

But the fact remains: not just Americans but all of us around the world are getting fatter, with an associated rise in type-2 diabetes, joint-related issues, etc. The number of artificial knee replacements in the US more than doubled to 615,000 in the ten years to 2008. According to UC Davis projections, knee and hip replacements will reach 4,500,000 by 2030.[99] OK, we have an ageing population, but our weight is clearly playing a role – combined with increased levels of arthritis, which in itself is an inflammatory disease associated in more and more scientific reports with diet-related problems. The American Arthritis Foundation recommends the benefits of a Mediterranean diet 'low in processed foods and saturated fat and rich in fruits, vegetables, fish, nuts and beans'.[100] Now ... where I have I seen that before?

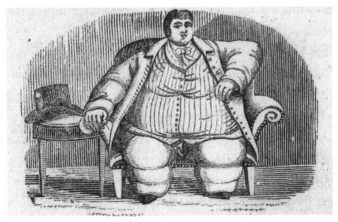

Figure 8:   Daniel Lambert weighed 50 stone (over 300 kilos) at the time of his death
             in 1809. He charged people money to see him in shows; a sign of how rare
             obesity used to be.

Things were very different two hundred years ago. On April 2nd, 1806 an advertisement in *The Times* newspaper described a Mr Daniel Lambert as 'the greatest Curiosity in the World who at the age of 36 weighs upwards of fifty stone'. That works out at over 300 kilos, but the funny thing about the ad was that it invited interested parties to visit him at his house in Piccadilly for the entry fee of one shilling. Apparently, Daniel Lambert had been fit and strong in his youth. But when he

99   Giordani, 2014.
100 Paturel, 2015.

succeeded his father as keeper at Leicester City gaol, he began to lead a sedentary life and quickly gained weight. After moving to London, he became quite wealthy because at the time he was truly unique. Being fat was both weird and highly unusual, so people really did pay for an audience with him. The *Leicester Mercury* described him in 1809 as 'one of the city's most cherished icons'. Sadly, he died – most probably from heart disease – at the age of 39.

The hormonal imbalance that led to Lambert becoming obese may have made him a 'curiosity in the world' two hundred years ago, but he would be one of many today. According to a report last year, Britain alone has more than a hundred thousand similar 'super-obese' people; those being defined as having a body mass index of above 50. To add a melancholy touch: if you are looking for a growing business, the market for super-sized coffins is literally expanding fast.

So, are we consuming more energy (calories) than we expend? In other words, all things being equal, are we still eating too much and moving too little? Another well-accepted stance is that when it comes to our appetite, we are at the mercy of those 'thrifty genes', which originally helped our survival by encouraging us to eat whenever food was available. Genetically, those of us alive today have survived because our ancestors were healthy and repetitive eaters capable of storing fat when needed. They were, in Darwin's terms, 'best adapted' to future possibilities, and the ancient (in evolutionary terms) hypothalamus in our brains still wants us to eat and store any surplus for those possible hard times that might just lie ahead. Our powerful biological drive to eat competes with a relatively weak appetite control system, which is why in restaurants it's hard to resist choosing a sweet dessert even when we are full.

After World War Two, when food rationing was the norm, governments led by the USA sponsored research and provided incentives which spurred on a true agricultural revolution. In their book, *Toward a Third Agricultural Revolution*, Wayne Rasmussen and Paul Stone refer to this phase as 'the application of chemistry to agricultural production'.[101] For most Westernised societies, it has meant that food is both more

---

101 Rasmussen and Stone, 1982, *Introduction*.

plentiful and much cheaper than it was in previous decades. In fact, the price of food has dropped from being over half of the household budget to less than 20% in Europe, and represents little more than 10% of the average American's take-home pay (although much of what is purchased would be classed as junk food). More recently, portion sizes have also increased – and that's not just with fast-food supersizing. Basic, small bags of crisps are twice as big as they were fifty years ago, and even plates and cups are around one-third larger in size. Just take a look at the average size of a coffee bought from your favourite shop these days. A caffé latte from Starbucks contains a full 16 ounces (just short of half a litre) of coffee.

And of course, similarly to what happened when Daniel Lambert took over his father's sedentary job, there is less physical effort involved in our daily routines. Labour-saving devices such as washing machines, driers and vacuum cleaners have resulted in an easier life, and cars are often used to travel short distances. In the past, physical activity was not a choice; it was simply a part of everyday life. The Rosetans, with their tightly knit community and Italian heritage, probably engaged in more walking around than some of their contemporaries.

Yet my eyes tell me something else. My brother runs a small hotel business and employs a number of people who actively work at washing and ironing, preparing the rooms and generally keeping things tidy. They are very active, burning up lots of calories while they work – but none of them are skinny. In fact, some are decidedly overweight – but I can probably guess what in their diet is causing this: an excess of carbohydrates.

Yes – if you eat too much, you will put on weight, and our super-sized society isn't helping. But the foods that you select will also impact your desire to eat, and as we have read, sugary foods, bread and other starches have a greater impact on your hormonal balance. Hormones play a big role in our thoughts, desires and actions. That's why it is wrong to simplify things and say that 'greed' or 'laziness' makes certain people fat. Simply eating more does not take into account the complex

145

physiological processes that control our behaviour and the role that what we eat has on determining our weight and body shape.

Dr Mackarness and a brief history of counting calories

In his 1959 book, *Eat Fat and Grow Slim*,[102] Richard Mackarness (a British doctor) exposed the 'calorie fallacy' and proposed a non-carbohydrate 'Stone Age' diet of protein and fat – with no restriction as to the amount eaten. Sounds way ahead of his time, with today's growing trend towards low-carb and paleo-style diets? Well, he certainly was. Dr Mackarness liked to use the very British analogy of a Rolls Royce motor car, which '… being the most expensive of cars, cannot clean its own pipes, clear its own choked jets, grind its own valves, re-line its own bearings when they are worn and replace defective parts as they need renewal'. We are, he determined when drawing the parallel to humans, so much more than just energy-burning machines; we maintain and repair ourselves along the way.

Indeed, we must remember that our bodies are clever at renewing themselves on a permanent basis. Red blood cells live for about four months, while white blood cells live on average for more than a year. Skin cells live for just two or three weeks, colon cells die off after about four days and sperm cells have a life span of about three days. Brain cells typically last an entire lifetime. Mackarness's book made reference to two distinct body types when considering how we maintain weight and/or diet: 'Mr Constant-Weight' and 'Mr Fatten-Easily'. Pertinently, he categorised himself within the second of these categories. The book was quite popular, particularly in the USA, and went through six editions – but the low-fat bandwagon which took over as the twentieth century progressed pushed his line of thought into the depths of obscurity. Only recently, with improved and more thoughtful scientific analyses, has his work enjoyed a small renaissance. Today, Dr Mackarness's book still provides refreshing and relevant insights.

---

102 Mackarness, 1959, p.57.

His particular way of dividing people into two groups according to the way they deal with excess food when they eat is, in many ways, still valid. He argued that two people of the same size, doing the same work and eating the same food will react quite differently when they over-eat. One will stay at about the same weight and the other will gain. It is worth pointing out that his references to 'Mr Constant-Weight' and 'Mr Fatten-Easily' might be updated today with a mix of genders. Yet today there is not just more gender awareness but more biological knowledge available, and so we can now alternatively position these two types of human being as being either 'hormonally happy' or 'hormonally challenged'.

The 'hormonally happy' Mr Constant-Weight has a more efficient body with an adaptable metabolic rate. The Constant-Weights can usually lose weight with any diet and often mix it with some exercise. As a group, they get closest to the supposed principles of calories in equalling calories out, but looking around us suggests that they are the exception rather than the rule.

On the other hand, the Fatten-Easilys are hormonally challenged and, being as a result more sensitive to insulin, they shift all too quickly into fat-storage mode. The ability to store food on your body is undoubtedly a trait that would have served them well in times of food shortage earlier in our evolutionary pathway, but today, it is helpful for no-one. At the time that Dr Mackarness wrote his book, food was again becoming plentiful after the war shortages. Now, with an abundance of cheap food, the possibility to over-eat is much greater than during those post-War times and the parallel to the Fatten-Easilys and their problems are all the more relevant.

An inherent problem with most guides to dieting is that they deal with everyone in the same way. Calorie restriction (that drop of usually 600 calories per day) means that the Fatten-Easilys (hormonally challenged) are deprived of good food and live with constant hunger, cheered on by their supporters as they lose weight in group motivation sessions (the Weight Watchers approach). The sad fact is that after leaving the semi-starvation diet and such groups of dietary friendship behind, they relapse and often end up weighing more than they originally did. That is how so many people find that the yo-yo approach to dieting begins to take over their lives. Somewhere in their late forties, they simply give up. In this light, it is perhaps not surprising that the highest proportion of obese people in the UK today is among the 45-54 age group, with about one in twenty-five being in the morbidly obese category and possessing a body mass index of above 40 (even allowing for the inaccuracies of BMI, readings of over 40 tell a clear story).

The simple problem with most dietary approaches is that they are prescribed by dieticians and nutritionists who have been taught that restricting calories creates a calorific deficit which leads to weight loss. The altar at which they worship is an equation named as 'energy balance', where eating and drinking are balanced against physical activity. Now, the facts do appear to support such an approach when it comes to the Constant-Weights (if and when they want to lose a pound or two). But for most of the rest of us, the Fatten-Easily majority, calorie restriction negatively affects our metabolic rate, causes mood-swings, results in a loss of energy and has little (if any) lasting impact on our weight loss.

Key points ...

1. Can we turn the Fatten-Easilys into Constant-Weights? Yes we can, but only if we attack the whole issue of diet in a different way, basing it on a hormonal approach and throwing the calorie-counting approach out of the window.

2. Back to 'calories in, calories out': according to the US Department of Agriculture,[103] in 1970 the food supply provided 2,086 calories per person per day, on average. By 2010, this amount had risen to 2,534 calories – an increase of more than 2% per year. Consuming an extra 448 calories each day should add nearly 25 kilos to the average adult in a year, they say. Well, if it had done that, Americans would have exploded a long time ago!

---

103 See earlier reference.

Is there too much 'nutritionism' in this calorie-controlled world?

Popularised by Michael Pollan (an American journalist and university lecturer) in his best-selling book, *In Defense of Food*,[104] Gyorgy Scrinis's concept of 'nutritionism' is used to refer to the reductive understanding of nutrients as the key indicators of healthy food. This approach now dominates nutrition science, dietary advice and food marketing around the world, and the calorie lies at its heart. Yet Michael Pollan argues compellingly that a food's nutritional value is:[105] 'more than just the sum of its parts'. As noted earlier, UK scientist and writer, Ben Goldacre, refers somewhat less diplomatically to nutritionism as the 'bollocks du jour', which is:[106] 'driven by a set of first year undergraduate errors in interpreting scientific data'.

Be that as it may, percentages of fat, protein and carbohydrate intake (together with their calorific values) drive most consumer thought when it comes to dieting and healthy eating these days. It's worth noting that the word 'calorie' has not really been around for that long and is a legacy of Napoleon's support for the introduction of the metric system. Originally defined in the 1845 edition of Bescherelle's French language dictionary, the word entered the English language in 1863 through the translation of Ganot's popular treatise on physics, which defined a kilo-calorie as the heat needed to raise the temperature of 1kg of water from 0 to 1°C. What we now refer to as everyday calories are in fact kilo-calories, and the capitalized 'Calorie' initiated by Atwater in 1887 indicates this in scientific papers. As such, you will often find calories with a big 'C' on today's food labels, though for easy readability when referring to calories, this book will use a small 'c'.

---

104 Pollan, 2008.
105 Pollan, 2007.
106 Goldacre, 2007.

If you visit the widely used online resource www.webmd.com, you can read a popular article which includes the quote: 'As far as <u>weight gain</u> is concerned, a calorie is a calorie,' from Lisa R. Young, PhD, RD, and author of *The Portion Teller Plan: The No Diet Reality Guide to Eating, Cheating, and Losing Weight Permanently*.[107] It reflects and supports the editorial viewpoint of www.webmd.com – and today's conventional wisdom in general – that you should start by reducing the quantity rather than first improving the quality of what you eat.

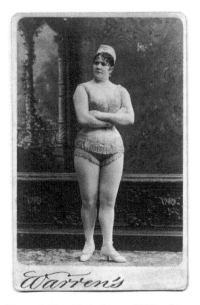

Figure 9: New York dancer, 1890 – this plumper body ideal was soon to change.

But, having read this far, aren't you too beginning to question whether it's quite as simple as that? Should our main focus really be directed at reducing the units of calorific energy?

In order to examine this topic further, we need to first provide a little additional historical context. When did calorie counting get started? How did we ever get to this calorific approach, and who will help us to understand why there is such a narrow focus on dieting? The broadly-based answer to the second question is 'women'; in particular, their shape and the objective and subjective perception of their figure.

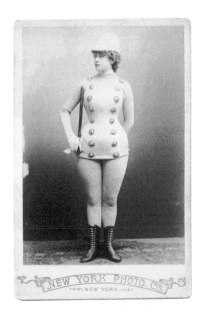

Figure 10: Burlesque dancer, Mlle Conalba – not the physique of today's dancers.

107 Kovacs, 2009.

It's fair to say that until the beginning of the twentieth century, Americans associated plumpness with beauty and wealth. Being too thin was often a sign of illness or poverty. The hourglass figure, with its corseted waist, full bust and wide hips, provided the role model in late Victorian times – though wearing a corset could cause both breathing and digestive problems.

But World War One was about to change all that. Women were to be found everywhere – in all lines of work – during the war. Correspondingly, both understanding and perception of their role in society began to change. A flatter-chested, narrow-hipped, long-legged figure became all the rage in the 1920s, and the flapper set, as they were known, brought in a fashionable slender physique as the ideal. These were rapidly changing times, with women winning the vote in 1920. The association with a slender physique also represented a certain social status; this look provided a kind of snob appeal, forming a visible difference between the working and the leisured classes. Dr Lulu Hunt-Peters was well-positioned to take advantage of this situation.

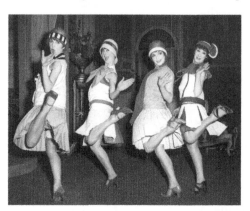

Figure 11: The flappers helped change women's role in society – and promoted a skinnier physique.

As a trained medical doctor who had earned her medical degree from the University of California in 1909 (itself unusual for a woman at the time), she could support and encourage new dieters by legitimising the promise of calorie counting with the necessary scientific understanding and background. She initially struggled with weight herself, and by telling her personal story about how she counted calories to become slim again she convinced millions to join her journey.

At her heaviest, Dr Hunt-Peters weighed 220 pounds (nearly 100 kilos). But she managed successfully to lose 70 of those pounds (just over 30 kilos) through reducing her calorie intake. With a view to the future, she accomplished this weight loss by collaborating with a group of like-minded friends. Her insistence that dieters re-imagine food as calories turned these calories into a kind of translatable language for a certain class of American society. But it must be noted that, although she was a doctor, her approach had little to do with health; it was all

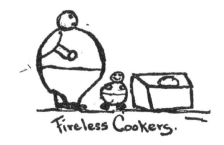

Figure 12: The body, seen as a food-burning furnace – from *Diet and Health* by Dr Hunt-Peters, 1918.

about female aesthetics. In fact, she paid scant attention to the type of foods a person should eat as long as they maintained a strict diet of 1,200 calories (for a person of her height) a day.

This was the period of real transformation from the calorie as a unit of heat value to the calorie becoming part of the body-shaping vocabulary. Hunt-Peters's book, entitled *Diet and Health: With Key to the Calories*,[108] was in continuous publication from 1918 to 1939 (and was re-issued in 2015). Although she died in 1930, she did more than anyone to establish the calorie as part of the new language of dieting.

Chemist Wilbur Olin Atwater had been the first to bring the scientific concept of the calorie to the United States after spending two years researching in Germany. As a 'Victorian with a solemn countenance', he pursued the study of the energy requirements of the human body at rest and in action; ironically, photos show that he was a bit on the tubby side himself. This was a time in the middle of the nineteenth century when scientists were just beginning to investigate the chemical composition of foods, and by the time we'd reached the 1920s, they had identified a host of vitamins and minerals considered essential for survival. The early focus was not on our dietary needs; the livestock industry was the first to express interest in measuring the heat energy contained in foods. Only later was this work scoped and further developed for humans. Until his death in 1907, Atwater wrote extensively about calories in *The Century* and in many US Department of Agriculture (USDA) publications,

---

108 Hunt-Peters, 1918.

explaining precisely what a calorie was and how many calories various foods contained. His estimates, published in 1888, were that[109] 'a woman with light exercise' required 2,300 calories per day, while an average man needed 2,830.

With the background of rapid industrialisation, physiologists and nutritionists argued that better nutrition would lead to healthier bodies and, in turn, more efficient workers. In turn-of-the-century Germany, the scientists began to examine human fatigue in terms of maximising productivity and the efficiency of labour. Meanwhile, in the United States, the emphasis turned to investigating calorie and nutrient requirements. Atwater was conducting dietary studies on bricklayers in Massachusetts to determine how many calories and grams of nutrients bricklayers required to perform their work. At roughly the same time, Frederick Taylor was promoting his famous highly analytical, factory time and motion studies. Taylor would break the work process down into its smallest possible units and determine the most efficient method for completing a particular job, while Atwater categorised different foods as if the body's job was simply to burn them.

The new gods of productivity and efficiency were taking over, and the calorie became an unlikely icon of this new era. It was effectively the introduction of food rationing during World War One by the Food Administration that first made the word 'calorie' commonplace. The government agency published numerous pamphlets which encouraged Americans to ration those foods shipped off to allied countries. This burgeoning familiarity with the word enabled Dr Lulu Hunt-Peters to use calories as the cornerstone of her diet success approach. The agency instructed Americans that they were in a position to ration food and still obtain enough calories. But by consuming more calories than recommended by the Food Administration's nutrition experts, they wrote, you were undermining the war effort. The first restaurant menus featuring calorie contents started appearing in New York City just over a hundred years ago and Americans steadily learned how to ration foods and find new substitutes where necessary.

109 See Jou, 2015.

Meanwhile, on the front line in France, the British Army attempted to give its soldiers the sum total of 3,574 calories a day; a figure that dieticians said was needed to keep them going. This number was, however, hotly disputed, with other voices arguing that soldiers during wartime needed much more than this. In the real world situation faced by those soldiers, it was generally a moot point; as the war progressed, the three hundred thousand or so staff of cooks and assistants struggled increasingly to meet their needs, resorting to scavenging and feeding them up on dishes such as locally sourced nettle soup. In spite of the 3,240,948 tons of food sent over from Britain to feed the soldiers fighting in France and Belgium during World War One, the bulk of it seemed to consist of bully beef (which is a type of canned corned beef), bread and biscuits, so much else being rationed or unobtainable.

When 1918 finally came, the war was over. Going back to post-war America, rationing was no longer needed. That is when Lulu Hunt-Peters began to address would-be American dieters. During this whole period of time, the compass needle swung slowly in the direction of fat as the primary target of dietary goals. This was primarily because fat carried twice the calorific punch as protein and carbohydrates. Where better to start with your dieting, said Dr Hunt-Peters.

Calorie counting went from strength to strength, supported later in the century by the increasingly strong US-led drive to reduce the amount of fat in your diet – this time for health reasons. It seemed like a 'win-win stuation'; being able to drop your fat intake to both lose weight and get healthy. But most of the evidence for the allegedly healthy contribution made by eating less fat was based on correlation and, as we know, correlation is not necessarily indicative of causation. Recent analyses of those earlier, influential studies have raised important questions about their validity, and revised government guidelines are now being considered in many countries.

Counting your calories does not always add up to the same figure, or so it seems. Estimating precise calorie levels turns out to be something of a can of worms, and in the 1970s researchers introduced modified Atwater values intended for specific food groups such as fruits, vegetables and beans. Since then, there have been very few changes – but their accuracy continues to be questioned. In 2012, researchers at the Human Nutrition Research Center in Beltsville, Maryland, found that almonds have 20% fewer calories than previously estimated.[110] According to the Atwater system, a one ounce (28 gram) serving of almonds has about 170 calories; but the researchers found that the energy content of the nuts was around 129 calories. One of the researchers (Baer) explained:[111] 'If we're going to put the information out there on the food label, it would be nice that it's accurate'. Famously, the Outback Steakhouse claimed their classic blue cheese wedge side salad had 376 calories, but lab results showed it had an impressive 1,035 when independently assessed. A separate study by the US Today show in the summer of 2014 found that so-called low-calorie ice creams and frozen yoghurts can contain as much as 68% more calories than the labels claim.[112]

Calorie counts also don't usually account for the fact that some calories in food are lost as heat – depending on the components of the food. For proteins, this can represent up to 30% of the food's calories, while for fats it is negligible. Researchers have recently discovered that twice-cooked potatoes (which have been cooled and then reheated) lose calorific value as more of the carbs are transformed into resistant starch.[113] The same goes for pasta and rice. There are also other inconsistencies. Most people don't seem to have a problem with all this as we've got used to quoting calorific values, and the situation is typically summed up as follows:[114] 'For most uses, I think they're good enough,' says Malden Nesheim, Professor Emeritus of Nutrition at Cornell University and co-author of the book *Why Calories Count*.[115]

This approach represents today's conventional wisdom. As for me, I don't look at calories any more although I do understand why they could help us in times of war or national emergencies. For day-to-day

110 Novotny et al., 2012.
111 Rettner, 2013.
112 Rossen and Powell, 2012.
113 Stoye, 2015.
114 Rettner, 2013.
115 Nestle and Nesheim, 2013.

living, they are at best an irrelevancy and a distraction – but people love to measure things, and that's an inherent part of the prolonged success of calories as the dieters' preferred yardstick.

For the record ... how do 'the experts' assess calorie levels?

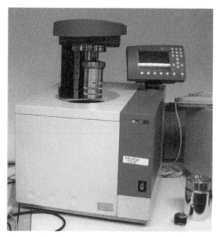

Figure 13: Please note the lack of similarity between a bomb calorimeter and the human digestive system.

Ever used a bomb calorimeter? A 'calorie' is a unit of energy transfer. We determine the number of 'calories' in any particular food by, quite literally, burning it and measuring how much heat it generates. Yet our bodies are not steam engines or motor cars. They do not burn the food we eat in a fire and then convert that heat into mechanical work. The metabolic pathway within our body begins with a specific molecule being converted into another molecule – usually consuming energy in the process, but not producing it.

That's why we need to eat food. As a result, we remain living. All those chemical reactions that build and repair each one of the trillions of cells in your body, from the top of your brain down to your big toe, require both energy and raw materials. The chemical reactions that allow our cells to perform all these different but necessary functions, from transporting oxygen to interpreting visual input to generating muscular force to manufacturing mucus, bile, stomach acid and insulin etc. require both energy and raw materials. And the chemical reactions that allow our cells to communicate, via hormones and neurotransmitters, also require both energy and raw materials. In summary, this is what really happens to the food we eat. It:

- builds and repairs our tissues, both cellular (e.g. muscles, skin, nerves) and acellular (e.g. hair, collagen, bone mineral).

158

- produces enzymes, hormones, and other molecules necessary for cellular function and communication.

- produces bile, stomach acid, mucus and other necessary secretions, both internal and external.

- is used by gut bacteria to keep them alive. The waste products of its metabolism can result in:

    o poor digestion, in which case it is at least partially excreted;

    o conversion into a form in which it can be stored for future use, such as glycogen or fat;

    o transportation to an individual cell, before conversion to energy, in order to perform any of the abovementioned tasks.

Looked at in the context of obesity and potentially shedding weight, only one point on this list can be seen as undesirable – that's the fat storage issue. To reduce the body's highly specialised and personal ecosystem and liken it to the way a furnace burns up food is simplistic at best and surprisingly naïve if you really think it through.

But for now, calories rule the roost. Even celebrity chefs (such as Jamie Oliver) who advocate a return to more home cooking end up using low-fat yoghurt in their recipes to bring the calorie count down. 'The benefit of choosing fruits, vegetables and other lower-fat foods is that you get more bang for your buck,' says Betsy Klein,[116] a Miami-based dietician quoted in *WebMD*, the world's second-most-visited health website. 'Carbohydrates and protein have 4 calories per gram, while fats have more than twice as much – an entire 9 calories per gram. If you're counting calories to lose weight but eating higher-fat foods like bacon and full-fat cheese, you could potentially consume over half your day's calorie allotment by the end of breakfast,' she says. 'Choosing carbs and protein for your morning meal, on the other hand, like an egg white

116 Kovacs, 2009.

159

omelette stuffed with mushrooms, onions, green peppers, and a small amount of low-fat cheese, will leave you with calories to spare for meals and snacks beyond breakfast.'

This all sounds so logical, doesn't it? But with fat playing such an important role in establishing your hormonal balance, how you digest foods, how you take up minerals and the absorption of vitamins and other nutrients, this over-simplistic approach just continues to lead us up the garden path.

Great-Grandma knew best

In the mid-1950s, an unlikely anti-hero emerged on the small British TV screen. Billy Bunter was his name, and Greyfriars was the fictional British school that he attended. Interestingly, Gerald Campion, who played the lead role, was already twenty-nine years of age when he took on the role of playing the original corpulent schoolboy. And corpulent he was. Obese, even by today's standards.

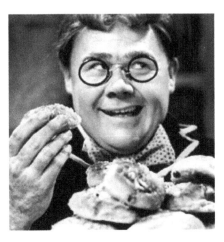

Figure 14: Billy Bunter – the 1950s TV star as portrayed by Gerald Campion.

According to Frank Richards (pseudonym), the author of the original books and comics, at fifteen years of age, Billy Bunter was 4 feet 9 inches tall and weighed 14 stone, 12 ½ pounds[117] – that's 1m 45 cm in height with a weight of almost exactly 95 kilos (in today's more familiar terms)!

In total, fifty-two half-hour episodes of Billy Bunter were broadcast between 1952 and 1961. As portrayed in these TV shows, apart from embodying most of the other seven deadly sins, he was particularly famous for his greed and gluttony. Obsessed as he was with food, he would eat as many of the stickiest, sweetest cakes and pastries as he could get his hands on, often helping himself to his schoolfellows' supplies. And had you asked anyone back in the 1950s what was making him fat, the answer would have been all too obvious: too many buns and cakes, too much jam and, probably, too little exercise. 'Everyone knows that,' your great-grandma would have said.

Yet today's 'conventional wisdom' has changed. When we treat overweight kids and adults today, a diet of low-fat food and low or

---

117 Richards, F. 1939.

no-fat milk is prescribed, and to put things right, we tell them to eat healthy grains. How our attitudes have changed! Let's look at how the carbohydrates and fats stack up. It's difficult to benchmark exactly what Billy Bunter ate, so here are some modern-day examples.

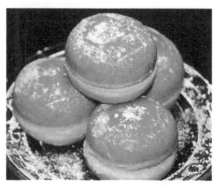

Figure 15: Just one of these cream doughnuts contains 51 grams of carbs, 27 grams of which is sugar.

According to www.fatsecret.co.uk, there are 8 grams of fat and 36 grams of carbohydrate (mostly flour and sugar) to be found in one portion of Mr Kipling apple pie. In one medium cinnamon bun, there are 9 grams of fat and 31 grams of carbohydrate. As to Billy Bunter's habit of eating spoonfuls of jam straight from the jar, each teaspoon of his favourite strawberry jam has 10 grams of carbs and no fat (*Tesco* jam is used as an example here). And, just to round it off, sponge cake with icing contains 5 grams of fat and 62 grams of carbohydrates per portion, more than half of which is sugar. For many years now, our use of sugar has grown and grown since it became cheaper and more widely available in the mid-nineteenth century. Apart from an understandable glitch during World Wars One and Two (see Figure 16), the rise continues although sweet syrup made from corn (HFCS on the food labels) now represents much of the 'sugar' we consume in prepared foods. Already, in 1985, Coca-Cola made the switch to using the cheaper 100 percent corn syrup in all its US based cola and non-cola drinks.[118] There is a slight taste difference though and rather mischievously to this day, there's a kind of black market for Mexican Coke - which is still largely sugar-sweetened - in the Southern States.

---

118 Elmore, 2015, Chapter 9: *High Fructose Corn Syrup*.

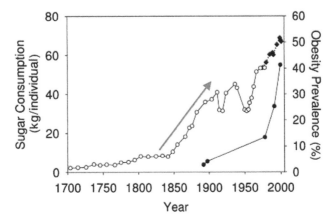

Figure 16: UK sugar consumption figures 1700-1978, with US figures for 1975-2000 added in black. Compare with obesity rates in US for those aged 60-69.

Going back to that portion of sponge cake, 62 grams is an awful lot of carbohydrates, and most comes in the form of the sweet stuff, be it sugar cane, beet or corn based. So the old-fashioned advice of telling young master Billy Bunter to stop eating sweet cakes and buns, was probably right on the ball – particularly when quantity enters the equation. But was it the fat or was it the carbs, or were they both combining to make him fat? Dr Ludwig, Professor of Pediatrics & Nutrition at the Harvard Medical School and founder of the Optimal Weight for Life programme (OWL), conducted (with colleagues) a relevant study at the Boston Children's hospital. The results of the study, published in 2012,[119] demonstrated pretty conclusively that children who have been first made to lose weight (i.e., with a drastically reduced food intake) maintained their new lower weight most easily on a carbohydrate-reduced diet because their metabolism sped up. He believes that it's the proportions of the different nutrients in your diet that can trigger weight gain if you get them wrong. Put more explicitly, even when protein levels are maintained, lowering carbohydrates and by definition increasing the amount of fat you eat will help you lose or maintain weight because your body becomes more efficient – you burn up your food more quickly, and you feel full faster.

---

119 Ebbeling et al., 2012.

These findings are in stark contrast to the earlier-mentioned 'conventional wisdom' of today, which says that because fats are more dense they add more calories and fatten you more easily. How simplistic is that! No wonder low-fat diets leave you feeling hungry and wanting the next snack.

So, where do the health authorities stand? In the UK, the National Health Service (NHS) website informs us in 2015 that:[120] 'Most adults in England are overweight or obese. That means many of us are eating more than we need, and should eat less'. It goes on to ask parents to 'lead by example and eat a balanced diet', which is defined in this way: 'A diet based on starchy foods such as potatoes, bread, rice and pasta; with plenty of fruit and vegetables; some protein-rich foods such as meat, fish and lentils; some milk and dairy foods; and not too much fat, salt or sugar, will give you all the nutrients you need'.

While it is true that the NHS is not advocating the consumption of sticky buns, they are replacing them with potatoes, bread, rice and pasta. It is the same NHS that features fast-food restaurants, snack bar shops and baguette bars in many of its hospitals. Yet the research by Dr Ludwig and colleagues showed us that a carbohydrate-rich diet, just as prescribed by the NHS, has a negative effect on our metabolism. It makes us burn food more slowly – not to mention the hormonal impact already covered. Could this be the real reason why, in spite of their advice, 'most adults are overweight or obese'? Perhaps it is because of their advice, most people are overweight or obese. This viewpoint is still controversial, I know, but it's worth thinking about. Admittedly, more studies are needed. But given where we are today, I think we all know that low-fat spreads and large quantities of starchy foods are not the way to go. Perhaps the folks at the NHS should read up on Billy Bunter. True, they would never have recommended his sugar fixation. But isn't it time they started recommending that we reduce the amounts of refined carbs? It appears that these things are really doing the damage, whether they are in the form of sugar, pizza, sliced bread or mashed potatoes.

---

120 NHS, 2015 (1).

I have previously made reference to Michael Pollan's insightful book, *In Defense of Food*, published back in 2008. This puts forward the notion that we are all victims of the ideology called 'nutritionism', which is based on several 'unexamined assumptions'. Among them is the assumption that 'foods are essentially the sum of their nutrient parts'. The research conducted by the team at the Boston Childrens' Hospital showed that such an over-simplistic approach just doesn't work. Michael Pollan also says:[121] 'Don't eat anything your great-grandmother wouldn't recognize as food'. Well, I hardly knew my great-grandmother, but I do remember my grandmother mentioning these words of advice when she was once asked about her slim figure: 'No snacks, no sweets, no seconds', she said. Surely appropriate for Mr Billy Bunter, too. But to stop the snacking, you need to first feel full; something that just doesn't happen for more than a short period of time when you're weaned on today's junk food and low-fat diets.

121 Pollan, 2006.

More about the role of the hormone, leptin

Leptin is the hormone produced by your body's fat cells; it is sometimes known as the fullness indicator. It can be administered externally in the form of pills or injections to induce weight loss,[122] but that belongs to the world of fringe medicine for now. Its primary target is a small part of the old (in evolutionary terms) brain called the hypothalamus, and apes and many other animals also use this indicator to tell them that they have enough stored fat and that they no longer need to eat. But for humans, things don't always work that way.

Leptin also impacts your immune system and certain brain functions, but its main role is in looking after your energy balance – how much you eat, how much you use and (of course) how much fat you store. As a hormone, it is carried in the bloodstream. When it reaches your brain, high levels indicate that there is sufficient stored fat, while low levels send a message that fat stores are getting low and you are at imminent risk of starvation. Although this hormonal system evolved to keep us from starving or over-eating, today something appears broken in the way it is supposed to prevent us over-eating. Put simply, it is not adapted to our world where most of us have easy access to relatively inexpensive food. In a nutshell, the system should function like this:

- When you eat, your body fat increases and your leptin levels go up. This means you eat less and draw on your fat reserves for energy when needed.

- If you don't eat, your body fat decreases and your leptin levels go down. This leads you to eat more and not use up too much of your fat reserves.

If you become overweight, you have an increased amount of body fat contained within your limited quantity of fat cells. Normally, unless you

---

122 Heymsfield et al., 1999.

are highly obese, you don't generate any more fat cells after puberty[123] In other words, if you put on weight, those fat cells just get bigger. As they will have increased their output of leptin, you should have stopped eating (or at least wanted to stop). Your brain should have recognised those signs, but if that leptin signal isn't getting through, something has gone wrong with the system. This 'malfunction' is now considered by many to be the root cause of human obesity. It is commonly known as leptin resistance. Because your brain doesn't pick up the leptin signal, it makes the mistake of thinking that you are still hungry – even though you have more than enough energy stored up in your fat cells. And there's another side to this as well. When your leptin levels go down or the receptors are no longer working efficiently, this doesn't just lead to you having an increased appetite level; it also reduces your general sense of get-up-and-go – your motivation to exercise.

Today's obesity drama is not caused by people's gluttony, laziness or lack of willpower. It is the biochemical, hormonal forces at play, and these are heavily influenced by our carb-rich, processed junk food diets. As we saw with the Pacific Islanders, wherever this Western diet becomes the norm, type-2 diabetes levels rise – as does obesity, however you care to measure it.

Our diet is not turning us into gluttons, but it is changing our very way of metabolising foods, forcing dramatic changes in lifestyle and behaviour. A simple but aggressive way of putting it goes like this: excessive amounts of refined carbohydrates, particularly sugar, are driving up our blood sugar levels. This in turn increases the secretion of insulin and results in us putting on weight in the form of fat storage. When leptin signalling no longer functions, our conventional doctors run out of ideas – and from this has grown the stomach stapling industry.

Of course, what constitutes 'excessive amounts of carbohydrates' can vary from person to person and may also depend on what type of carbs we are talking about. Two examples: young, fit men often tolerate a lot of carbs, even sugar, without gaining much weight, but middle-aged obese women with type-2 diabetes do not.

123 Spalding et al., 2008.

Nevertheless, reducing your intake of carbs does bring about weight loss and helps you to gain energy. Although not everyone agrees about why or even how exactly low-carb dieting works, all seem to agree that it does work. Some will say that the easy weight loss in the first couple of weeks is more about losing a proportion of the water in your body. But even if that is so, it's not really the point, because being lighter makes you feel better.

Liver problems? You may be skinny on the outside but fat inside

Let's not get too hung up on being overweight. After all, a little extra weight does not seem to have harmed the inhabitants of Roseto. There's a well-visited TED talk given by Peter Attia,[124] who tells his personal story of encountering diabesity as a fit and athletic person. He questions whether it is the pathway to diabesity (or insulin resistance, as it's more widely known), which really causes obesity. In so doing, he potentially turns things on their head. We are conditioned to believe these days that getting fat in itself is the leading cause of diabetes. Could we be looking at things upside down?

You could also watch the 2014 film, *Carb-Loaded*,[125] which documents how Lathe Poland faced up to the news that, as a slim, athletic person in his early thirties, he too had acquired type-2 diabetes. He likens it to fat, but on the inside. The film's title (aka the problem with his diet) is probably a bit of a give-away, but it brings to life the journalistic journey he took around the world, talking to many experts on health and nutrition as he tried to find what cause his diabetes – and a cure. Another recent film is *Sugar Coated*.[126] This features a compulsive Canadian athlete in his twenties who discovered that he too was type-2 diabetic – mainly because of all the sugar he was eating and quite independent from his strict regimen of exercising. You could use these cases as pointers indicating that excess carbs (in particular, sugars) are what's driving this disease. You could be right; you could be wrong. And herein lies the problem.

Doctors and nutritionists disagree on what constitutes healthy food, and trained dieticians usually follow what they've been taught in their CW (Conventional Wisdom)-based courses – that being the low-fat

---

124 TEDMED, 2013.
125 TheSceneLab, 2014.
126 The Cutting Factory, 2015.

diet/more exercise mantra. Such an approach has certainly not helped us on our pathway to where over one-third of Americans are considered in a pre-diabetic stage, with the rest of the world showing every sign of wanting to catch up. A food's nutritional value, argues the acclaimed food writer Michael Pollan, is far more than the sum of its parts.[127] Yet our trained advisors coerce us with precise levels of macronutrients, supplements in the form of pills and powders and whey shakes made from the by-product of milk we are advised not to drink because it's not natural. Whatever happened to real food, you might well ask.

There is now enough evidence that obese people are not the only ones facing future health issues and medical problems. One in four skinny people in the USA also have pre-diabetes, better known as insulin resistance – so this new disease (which simply did not exist one hundred years ago and is on its way to conquering the rest of the world) must be considered highly infective. Its means of infection? The highly processed Western diet. That's right; the countries with the highest levels of diabetes have exported their foods and eating habits to the healthier countries and we can measure the spread of the disease by what it's doing to our livers – and what it will soon be doing to theirs. Thinking back to our hormonally well-balanced Mr Constant-Weight; perhaps he too is on his way to getting fatty liver disease if he eats too much junk food – and particularly processed carbs.

Say 'liver disease' out loud to a group of people in a room and the first word that comes off their lips is almost universally 'alcohol' – an excess of it, that is. Non-alcoholic fatty liver disease (NAFLD) is still relatively unknown, but it has crept up on us and has now reached epidemic proportions in many Westernised countries. According to Dr Quentin Anstee (a liver specialist at Newcastle University),[128] although we have long associated liver damage with alcoholism, over-eating is now 'neck and neck' with drinking as a cause. And he predicts it will soon be the main trigger of fatty liver disease, just as it has become in the USA.

---

127 Pollan, 2007.
128 The Guardian, 2015.

Part of our problem in comprehending this is that NAFLD is not caused by eating too much fat. Whereas alcohol plays the single lead role in driving alcoholic liver disease, over-eating in general is seen here as the culprit – with excess calories being stored as fat in the liver. An article on the American Liver Foundation website, written by Dr John Goff, tells us that about 30% of US citizens now have NAFLD.[129] The American Liver Foundation's take on it is that 'NAFLD tends to develop in people who are overweight or obese or have diabetes, high cholesterol or high triglycerides. Rapid weight loss and poor eating habits also may lead to NAFLD'.[130] A disease of decadence, if ever I saw one! There appears to be no easy target or buzzword like the role which alcohol plays in the older, more established version of the disease. Over-eating signals an excess in all foods, but – as with the whole 'calories in, calories out' argument – we need to talk about quality and not just quantity. To fix things and start tackling this serious liver disease with any reasonable chance of success, that's what needs to change.

It may well be true that suffering from NAFLD has a high correlation with obesity. But now that more people are suffering from this newer form of fatty liver disease than are having their livers ruined by an excess of alcohol, should we simply be putting it down to over-indulgence? Could stress or other reasons play a role, or does simple and straightforward evidence point the finger firmly at our junk food diets and in particular to a surplus of carbs in our diet?

Answering this is critical because you really do want to look after your liver. It's an incredible organ and – if treated well – will easily outlast your body. It is one of the organs that can even be used to transplant into younger people in need; yes, even if you are a much older donor than the organ receiver. Your liver typically ages well, but only if you treat it with some respect. Let's look for further clues by seeing what WebMD has to say; after all, that website has over 156 million unique visitors per month (as of Feb 2014). It states:[131] 'Some fat in your liver is normal. But if it

---

129 Goff, 2012.
130 American Liver Foundation, 2015.
131 WebMD, 2014.

makes up more than 5-10% of the organ's weight, you may have fatty liver disease. If you're a drinker, stop'.

And that's the standard, puritanical message from doctors and health authorities everywhere. But maybe it's time to start updating the message, since NAFLD already exceeds the alcohol-related kind and is the most common liver disorder in Western industrialised countries.[132]

If you have NAFLD, at least no-one disputes the main symptoms. These include feeling tired, weight or appetite loss, weakness, nausea – even confusion, poor judgement and trouble in concentrating. But the remedy cited by *WebMD*,[133] 'Eat a balanced and healthy diet and get regular exercise', is pretty bland – and, as we know, it means different things to different people. To be fair, they have now added a recent update suggesting that you should be limiting high-carb foods as well as drinks containing sugar. But here's the thing: more and more evidence tells us that this should be message number one. A study published in April 2015 in the Hepatobiliary Surgery section of the US National Library for Medicine refers to fructose as[134] 'a weapon of mass destruction'. We need to be telling people that by drastically reducing their intake of carbohydrates, particularly sugar, they can increase their chances of keeping a healthy liver right into old age. Just as the abuse of alcohol leads in many cases to liver disease, so does a steady excess of carbohydrates.

In a Harvard Health Letter from 2011,[135] reference is made to fatty liver disease as a disease which: '… used to occur almost exclusively in people who drink excessively'. They start by saying: 'The epidemics of obesity and diabetes are to blame', but go on to say '… we are generally led to believe that being overweight is unhealthy and if we are thin, then we are healthy. But new research points to just how dangerous being skinny can be – if you are a skinny fat person, that is'.

This provides us with yet another indicator that our diets are affecting all of us; even those who look 'good' from the outside. In fact, a 2012

---

132 Sheth and Chopra, 2015.
133 WebMD, 2014.
134 Basaranoglu et al., 2015.
135 Harvard Health Publications, Harvard Medical School, 2011.

study showed that:[136] 'Adults who were normal weight at the time of incident diabetes had higher mortality than adults who are overweight or obese'. Don't get me wrong; obesity is not generally a good thing – it weighs down on our joints (quite literally) as well as increasing our chance of various diseases. But … it may not be the driver of diabetes that we think it is. It may be just part of the problem. Although unproven, Dr Attia may well have it right when he questions whether the pathway to insulin-resistance, which is so richly strewn with processed carbs of all kind, is really at the heart of the problem. Maybe it's not the obesity causing the diabetes, but the carbs. And if, like most of us, you're in the 'Fatten-Easily' camp, you get fat.

There are people who never seem to gain weight yet eat diets rich in bread, pasta and sugar. You may well know some, just as you may know some smokers who don't seem to be affected – yet what's happening to them on the inside? Their spiking insulin levels are also leading to hormonal and metabolic changes that cause muscle loss and inflammation and over time can lead to type-2 diabetes. They just don't show it because their hormones work differently. Maybe we have reached a time when we need to change our viewpoint. Let us consider that when it comes to insulin resistance and your liver, it's not a matter of whether you are skinny or fat, it's a matter of what you eat.

What this means is that to keep a healthy liver and avoid the pathway that leads to type-2 diabetes, your dietary and lifestyle guidelines should be the same, whether you are slim, overweight or obese. Consider these guidelines:

1. Don't drink sugar: avoid sodas, fruit juices and sweetened drinks. If taking alcohol, stick to small quantities of dry wine or spirits.

2. Avoid flour, including whole-grain and gluten-free flour products.

3. Eat animal protein, dairy, nuts, seeds, beans, vegetables (primarily from above the ground) and berries.

---

136 Carnethon et al., 2012.

4. Avoid processed and pre-packaged foods wherever you can.

5. Increase your intake of omega-3 fat rich foods such as sardines, mackerel and salmon; flaxseeds and walnuts; basil and spinach; and outside-reared and free-range meats and eggs.

6. Avoid refined and processed seed-oils made from corn, soy, sunflower etc. and increase your use of butter, lard, beef tallow, coconut and olive oil. Duck and goose fat are fine, too.

7. If our diet is healthy, most of us do not need supplements – unless you don't get enough sunlight, in which case extra vitamin D is essential.

8. Protect your body clock and exercise gently: if your working day (and geographic location) allows, sleep when it's dark, rise with the sun. Your circadian rhythm demands no better.

The danger signs: when it comes to insulin resistance/diabesity, too many carbs lead you to have regularly high levels of blood sugar circulating – hence the extra insulin getting pumped into your bloodstream. What happens then is that your muscle, fat and liver cells stop responding normally to that insulin building up in your blood. The chances that you will become diabetic and also have heart disease rise progressively as your liver continues to increase the amount of free fatty acids circulating in the blood (you'll register that as higher triglyceride levels and more LDL – 'bad cholesterol', for example).

The fattened cells in your liver lead to inflammation and can then go on to damage the surrounding liver tissue. This represents the start of a cascade of problematic damage to your liver. This eventually leads to cirrhosis, which is sadly irreversible, and to an increased risk of liver cancer.

Yet you should know that your liver is very resilient; in fact, your heart might give way before your liver. An article first published in

The New England Journal of Medicine in late 2009[137] and reviewed in the Harvard Health Letter argued that the inflammatory and other factors pumped out by a fat-afflicted liver promote the atherosclerotic process that damages the walls of arteries and makes blood more likely to clot – a combination that can lead to heart attack or stroke. Whatever happens exactly, it's not good news.

---

137 Harvard Health Publications, Harvard Medical School, 2011.

PART 6

WHAT YOU EAT AND HOW IT AFFECTS YOUR BODY AND YOUR DIGESTION

Interested in more detail?

If you have read this far, you will have built up a good degree of knowledge about what we eat and how it affects us. This next part is designed for those of you who want to dive a little deeper and effectively save some time when searching the Internet – or maybe even before considering whether to start a course in nutrition. Yes, while writing this book, I did indeed follow an online course and qualified at Level 5 within the UK Qualifications Framework. Apparently, 'Learning at this level involves the achievement of a high level of professional knowledge and is appropriate for people working as knowledge-based professionals or in professional management positions'. But, to be frank, I had to lie my way through some of the answers to pass the exam. Steeped in today's conventional wisdom, today's nutrition diplomas certainly do not allow for concepts such as 'fat is good for you' or accept that 'low-carb diets are the best way to treat diabetes'. To be sure of passing, I even had to tick the box that advised eating margarine over butter when dealing with weight loss. That was painful, but I did it to complete my certification!

An over-reliance on the analysis of macro- and micro-nutrients can lead to the kind of navel-gazing 'nutritionism' mentioned earlier. But a certain understanding of how our bodies digest such nutrients and the associated effects on our bodies will help us to understand the bigger picture. So here goes…

Protein, carbs and fat

The stomach's ability to digest and absorb nutrients varies wildly. When it comes to energy-rich proteins such as those found in meat, they are quite easy to digest. Others, such as the prolamins found in grains like wheat and corn, are poorly digestible; even after much effort, part of them will either linger on to feed our gut bacteria or be excreted. Once any protein is absorbed, its composition of amino acids will determine how much will be used for building and repair work, how much must be burned for energy and how much will be simply disposed of. Protein is an important building block for the body, but too much is too much. Even when the protein you eat is perfectly digested, if you have already absorbed enough complete protein for your daily needs and your exercise needs don't require additional muscle build, what's left over will still be converted into glucose, burned for energy or excreted – even if it is of the very highest quality.

Referring to the 'calories in, calories out' context, it's easy to see that a calorie of meat protein used to build muscle cannot equal a calorie of protein which is surplus to your needs. And in no way does it equal a calorie of partially digested wheat protein, which may be still disrupting your digestive tract.

These days, we generally live with an excess of readily available food, and our drive to consume is no longer driven principally by hunger but by an almost addictive sense of desire. That desire is fed by a surplus of quick-burning carbohydrates typified by those found in table sugar, which is a blend of 50% glucose and 50% sucrose. When you eat a spoonful of table sugar, your digestive system will use enzymes to break down the sucrose into its individual sugar units of glucose and fructose. Your body also processes most of the carbohydrates you eat into glucose, which is also called blood sugar, since small amounts circulate in the blood. Glucose is then either used immediately for energy, stored in muscle cells or in the liver as glycogen for later use, or – more often than not – used for fat synthesis and storage. That is the process which is stimulated by the insulin released in response to your glucose (blood sugar) levels.

Let's look at what happens to you when you eat 100 calories of fructose (fruit sugar), which is pure carbohydrate.

First, the fructose enters your liver from the digestive tract. It is turned into glucose and initially stored as glycogen.[138] But wait; your liver has a limited storage capacity, so if it is already full of glycogen, excess glucose is then turned into fat and effectively sent to the body's storage department – unless, that is, it is able to temporarily increase the size of your liver. When this process is repeated many times over days, months and then years, it is likely to lead to fatty liver disease. That excess of fructose is what leads to insulin resistance, which raises insulin levels all over your body, driving further fat gain. Added to this, fructose does not trigger your sense of fullness. This is because it has no effect on the hunger hormone ghrelin or the satiation hormone leptin – it is not registered by your body's internal organs in the same way as glucose is. Just for the record, the sugar used in today's manufactured foods is now often the cheaper processed high-fructose corn syrup, which is supposed to be no more than 55% fructose – though research from October 2010 found that it often exceeded that level.[139]

In a nutshell: when you eat 100 calories of fructose, your insulin levels increase over the long term – yet you continue to feel hungry. Let's compare that to what happens when you eat 100 calories of protein.

Protein uses up more energy during the digestive process, so about 30% of the initial calories will first of all be spent on digestion. The protein contributes to an increased level of fullness and, as an added plus, increases your metabolic rate. It goes on to be used in building muscles (as long as you've not eaten too much for your needs) and as active tissue. These continue to use up energy as and when you use them – as opposed to fat, which generally just sits around.

---

138 See Campbell and Farrell, 2015, Section 18–1.
139 Ventura et al., 2010.

Your hormones begin to signal a feeling of fullness after fifteen minutes or so, but the whole process of digestion can take around forty hours, so getting all the nutrients from the food you eat is important. When it comes to fat, proper digestion requires that your gastro-intestinal tract, liver, gallbladder and pancreas all work in harmony, and they usually do so amazingly well.

The digestion of fat begins in the mouth. First, it is broken down into smaller pieces by your teeth as they grind the food you eat. Then, early chemical digestion begins as your saliva moistens and emulsifies the fat, making it easier to swallow. It is then further broken down in your stomach until it takes on a semi-liquid form known as chyme. This proceeds onward to the small intestine where nutrients are absorbed and the real breakdown or digestion of fat takes place. Because fats do not dissolve in water, bile secreted by the liver prevents it all clogging together. Lipases break down the fat molecules into fatty acids and mono-glycerides, which pass through into the small intestine. These fatty acids are converted to triglycerides, which combine with cholesterol, phospholipids and protein to form a structure called a chylomicron whose protein coating makes it water-soluble so it can travel on through the lymph vessels and eventually the bloodstream. Doctors will analyse our blood readings by calculating the number and size of these tiny structures and itemising them as LDL or HDL, for example.

How full you feel after you have begun to eat plays a big role in dieting and general health. Try cooking and eating a protein and fat-rich three-egg omelette and then follow it up with another. After some time, you will feel full, and that feeling stays around for several hours. Yet I'm sad to confess that I have seen one of my sons down a half-litre of (fructose-rich) vanilla ice cream, following it up a couple of hours later with more food. Triggering the right hormones to remind your body that you are not hungry is essential if you want to have a healthy body and reach your targeted set-point. Commercial ice cream, like many other processed foods, also uses cheap high-fructose corn syrup (HFCS) as its principal sweetener. As you have read, this contains even more fructose than you find in regular sugar. It's yet another effect of the subsidies still going out to maize growers in the USA – cheap fructose that's damaging our bodies.

This all leads to a key difference between two very different dietary approaches – namely the prevalent low-fat diet or one based on lowering your carb intake and increasing the amount of fat you eat. Whereas people on low-fat diets need calorie restriction to lose weight, people eating low-carb (and correspondingly higher fat) food can usually eat until they feel satisfied and still lose weight. A number of research studies have shown that low-carb dieters begin to consume fewer calories simply because they feel full and their appetite goes down.[140] When you remove sugar and starch from your diet, it initiates a kind of chain reaction which stabilises blood sugar. The resulting lower level of insulin increases your body's ability to burn fat. This, in turn, makes you feel less hungry.

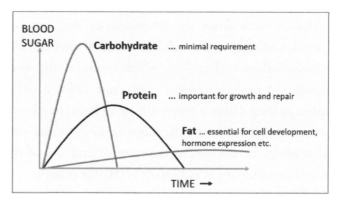

Figure 17:   If someone were to create a drug as effective as the slow-burning nature of eating fat ...

This all has to do with the concept of fullness. That three-egg omelette I referred to earlier is rich in protein and fat. Whether one is enough or whether you try to eat a second one, your sense of fullness will last for several hours. This is not the case when you eat as many carbs as the average person does on a conventional Western diet. You feel hungry again after a hearty breakfast, and you may also feel like a nap in the afternoon because of the effect of the insulin/blood sugar curve. This

---

140 See Foster et al., 2010.

curve also provides impetus to the huge snack industry – our craze for snacking is a direct result of short-term carb overloads.

As for me, I have never been on a calorie-restricted diet that has satisfied me. That was Katy's experience too. And we are certainly not alone.

The thing is: going hungry is effectively a form of continuous starvation. This is one of the main reasons that I now question calorie-controlled diets – that and the resulting imbalance of healthy nutrients caused by too few oils and fats. Fasting for a day here and there is another matter; it is quite different from reducing your food intake every single day over weeks. There is growing evidence that occasional fasts can help people lose or maintain weight, but this won't help if you have already been eating too many carbs for years and suffer – as so many people do – from insulin resistance.

Carbohydrates may fill you up, at least temporarily, but they do nothing to ease your longer-term hunger pains. That explains why counting calories but still eating a high proportion of carbohydrates (even if you do lose some weight) is less efficient than being on a low-carb diet – it's also less satisfying and generally more difficult to stick to.

This also explains why my son can eat that half-litre (500g) of ice cream in one go but would struggle to eat half a kilo of steak – even though it has many fewer calories. Eating carbohydrates spikes the blood sugar and leads you to want more a couple of hours later, while protein or fat consumption both release glucose into the system on a steadier basis over time. By cutting down your consumption of carbs, you can carry on eating without concern for calories – at least within reason. As we will discover later, finding the right (but lower than where you are today) proportion of carbs to everything else you eat is the true secret to weight loss and to eliminating any early indications of type-2 diabetes.

Coming back to today's world, the counting of calories still rules. Well-intentioned governments try to persuade fast-food outlets to put the number of calories on all their menu items, and even smaller restaurants are encouraged to do the same. This example of nutritionism often goes further, with the complete listings of all macro-ingredients, vitamins and trace elements also included – just like on food packaging. But just as vitamins in the form of pills will not always provide as many benefits as those found in real food, the nutrients in a pre-prepared shepherd's pie will not equate to the many benefits of preparing your own from fresh ingredients; especially when you consider the various preservatives, emulsifiers and colourants that are also in the commercially prepared products, and even if they do all contain roughly the same number of calories.

How junk food is changing your microbiome

Studies in lab mice have demonstrated that when fed an intensive high-fat, high-sugar diet, their microbes change dramatically and for the worse.[141] This can be partly prevented by adding probiotics, but there are obvious differences between us and lab mice, apart from our respective natural microbes – so is this research relevant for humans?

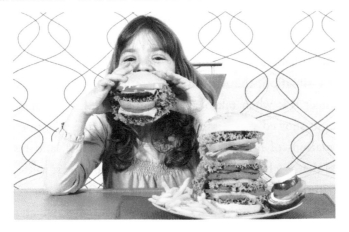

Figure 18:   Carbohydrates are the main ingredients in junk food.

In 2014, a study was conducted which focused on a group of rural Africans who ate a traditional local diet featuring beans, fruit and vegetables.[142] The study swapped their diet with that of a group of African-Americans who ate a high-fat, high-protein diet of sausages, hash browns, burgers and fries. This diet was, by definition, also low in dietary fibre. Just for the record, if this diet had been labelled 'Western junk-food diet' rather than 'high-fat', it would have been a more accurate label – but we're simply so used to labelling 'bad' food as 'high-fat'. The so-called high-fat Western diet was listed at 35% fat (or 15% by weight), which is not particularly high-fat at all. We can also assume that the fat and protein was not of the best quality, coming from CAFO

141 Oregon State University, 2015.
142 O'Keefe et al., 2014.

(Concentrated Animal Feeding Operations)-raised animals. (If this topic piques your interest, by the way, there is much more on the subject of CAFOs in a book entitled *The Tragedy of Industrial Animal Feeding Factories*, by Daniel Imhoff.[143]) The temporary Western diet in the study was also high in omega-6 fatty acids from fried seed oil – and, of course, high in refined and processed carbs, which also equates to low in fibre.

'We made them fried chicken, burgers and fries,' said Stephen J. D. O'Keefe, a gastroenterologist at the University of Pittsburgh and one of the study's authors.[144] 'They loved it.'

Yet in spite of their 'love' for the Western fast food, the Africans fared poorly on their temporary diet. Their metabolism changed, presenting a diabetic and unhealthy profile within just two weeks. In the reverse situation, the African-Americans showed lower markers for colon cancer risk when taken away from the junk food diet. Tests of both groups showed very different microbiomes (the scientific term for the populations of microbes contained in their guts), and researchers suggested that the higher fibre content played the biggest role.

One important difference which is not explained in the research is that the Africans were, in reality, put on a 52% fat diet, which will have distorted the results somewhat since my hunch is that the processed carbs are doing more damage than the classically trained researchers suspected. The rural African high-fibre diet led to gut microbes which produced more butyrate, a chemical with anti-cancer properties, while the Western diet meant that the microbes produced more bile acids, which can lead to an increased cancer risk.

Were the results more to do with a switch from refined carbs to the more natural carbs found in the beans, fruit and veggies? Did fat play a role? As with so much research in the field of nutrition, we cannot be sure – though it's clear that the American junk food diet is not helping anyone. It is also clear that we have more control over our individual health than some of the 'it's all in your genes' advocates would suggest. Jeremy Nicholson, a senior co-author on the study who is based at

---

143 Imhoff, 2010.
144 O'Keefe et al., 2014.

Imperial College, said: 'What is startling to me is how profoundly the microbes, metabolism and cancer risk factors change in just two weeks of diet change. It means to me that diet and environment and microbial genes are likely to be much more important than individual human genes in determining individual colonic cancer risks. Certainly it shows that your possible fate is not just determined by the genetic dice at birth. How you roll the dice in the game is probably more important'.

There are many anecdotal reports of the effects associated with eating junk food. Morgan Spurlock famously 'super-sized' himself for the documentary *Supersize Me*,[145] in which he gained weight, damaged his liver and claimed to have suffered addictive withdrawal symptoms. But (with the exception of this American/African study) when it comes to our microbiome, no-one – as yet – seems to have examined the effect that junk food may be having. With this in mind, Tim Spector (as he reports in his book *The Diet Myth: The Real Science Behind What We Eat*)[146] got his son, Tom (after much self-experimentation), to alter his diet and track his microbes as they changed. Tom went from what his father refers to as an average Western diet to an intensive fast-food diet for a week. His plan was to eat all his meals at McDonalds for a ten day period. The meals consisted of the usual suspects: Big Macs, chicken nuggets, French fries and non-diet Coca-Cola. As a treat – and to get some extra vitamins – beer and crisps were also on the menu each evening. Tom's temporary diet had made him physically unwell, but it took a few months for the results to arrive back. The results – which came from Cornell University in the US – showed to what extent Tom's microbiome had been devastated. According to Tom's father, the clearest marker of an unhealthy gut is losing species diversity. During these ten days, Tom had lost an estimated 1,400 species representing nearly 40% of his total gut bacteria. This represents an unambiguous signal of ill health and mirrors the limited number of bacteria found in the guts of many obese and diabetic people. Such a reduced content has also been shown to be a pre-cursor to immunity problems in laboratory mice.

---

145 2004.
146 Spector, 2015, Chapter 2: *Energy and Calories*.

Although this result is clearly not statistically representative, it does indicate that those who eat fast food on a regular basis are weakening their bodies' natural defences by reducing gut diversity. This leads Professor Spector to claim that a diet encouraging the growth of a range of gut bacteria might be as effective for weight loss as simply cutting back on macro-ingredients such as fat and sugary carbs. To accelerate this process, he suggests the following dietary supplements – celery, chicory root, garlic, cheese made from raw milk (unpasteurised), 85% dark chocolate and naturally brewed Belgian beer. Coffee also makes his good list, although it is a little further down the table.

Junk food rules today because it's cheap, convenient and tasty. The manufactured snack bars, burgers and so on are put together in a way that almost short-circuits our taste buds; their chemical concoction of sweet, aromatic and spicy additives are designed to get as close as possible to making us addicts. Junk food is cheap because the industrial subsidies that still encourage the use of its main ingredient, processed carbohydrates, are not factored into the price – and neither, of course, is a contribution towards the health costs which are needed to help you along the way when you eat a lot of fast food. Imagine there was a 20% health tax on junk food to help pay for your long-term medical bills. With cereal crops being subsidised to produce high-fructose corn syrups, starches and intensive animal feeds, unsubsidised fruit and vegetables in the market look more expensive than a fair comparison would allow. The sad fact is that Big Food is subsidised and tax-advantaged over Real Food.

The sugary, fatty combinations of refined and processed flour with all their emulsifiers, colourants and other additives are served up together with carbonated drinks in more and more countries around the world. Yet, in column inches, saturated fat in the form of butter, lard, coconut oil and others still gets the bulk of the blame for our diseased world. And if you were running Coca-Cola or Nestlé, you'd want to keep that 'fat is evil' message going just as long as you could.

Carbs, processed foods, emulsifiers and additives

Inevitably, some people ask me whether I've simply got something against carbohydrates. The answer is: no. The problem (as I see it) is that most people seem to think carbs are totally innocuous. This leads them to focus on 'bad' fat and 'good' protein to balance their 'healthy' diets. They don't even consider that the main harm in their diets today is being done to them by carbs ... not all carbs, I stress to add, but what I call 'fake-carbs' – together with a growing number of additives and preservatives.

These fake-carbs are namely the processed ones, which are mostly to be found in bottles, tins (cans for our American readers) packets and boxes. They are heavily refined foods that have usually been combined and modified in such a way as to create something highly edible, often sweet (although the sugar is often hidden) and definitely marketable. Their manufacturing process has changed them so that they usually bear little resemblance to the original ingredients – think 'Froot Loops', 'Frosted Flakes' or supposedly healthy 'muesli' bars, which are all rich in sugar. To preserve them and increase shelf life by many months, manufacturers used to add trans fats, which have now more or less been banned – so recently, they have upped the level of emulsifiers. Egg yolk is a natural emulsifier (thickener of oils). But of course, it doesn't add to shelf life; just think how home-made mayo will keep for just a few days in the fridge, whereas Hellman's will keep for months. So the manufacturers turn to synthetic emulsifiers you'll find listed as E-numbers in the 400 range, such as E480 (Dioctyl sodium sulphosuccinate) or E436 (Polyoxyethylene-20-sorbitan tristearate). These synthetic and semi-synthetic emulsifiers are in everything these days, from chewing gum to ice cream to processed meats.

According to the European Food Emulsifiers Manufacturers Association (EFEMA), the current world production of food emulsifiers is estimated at around 400,000 tonnes, comprising of some twenty types. Their website cites these key benefits:[147]

- Provides a stable, low-fat dressing without compromising taste or shelf life.

- Gives chewing gum its soft, chewy properties.

- Contributes a delightfully soft but not doughy crumb to bread.

We need to be concerned about what happens when we ingest these substances. Inflammatory bowel diseases are linked to a change in our gut microbiota (we each have something like 100 trillion of them in our intestines) which promotes various forms of inflammation. Dr Andrew T. Gewirtz of Georgia State University is a member of a team currently investigating the suspicious effects of emulsifiers on our digestive systems. He states (in a press release):[148] 'A key feature of these modern plagues (such as Irritable Bowel Syndrome) is alteration of the gut microbiota in a manner that promotes inflammation. Emulsifiers are a good candidate because they are so ubiquitous and their use has roughly paralleled the increase in these diseases'.

Interim results show that:[149] '... the current means of testing and approving food additives may not be adequate to prevent use of chemicals that promote diseases driven by low-grade inflammation and/or which will cause disease primarily in susceptible hosts'.

Questions are not just raised by the inclusion of various emulsifiers in ingredient lists but also by the stressful way carbohydrates are crushed, stretched, steamed and literally exploded in the production processes of today.

Consider, if you will, a flake of corn. When John Harvey Kellogg first invented the corn flake, it consisted more or less of a flattened

---

147 EFEMA, 2015.
148 Georgia State University News, 2015.
149 Idem.

individual grain of corn, dried and toasted to make it crispy – you can still try making them that way at home. But for many decades now, industrialised corn flakes have been produced by extruding a small piece of mushy boiled-up corn paste, shooting it into hot dry air to firm it up and then spraying it in a light mist of sugar to 'improve' the taste and help preserve the crispiness (that part is thanks to Kellogg's brother, William). Well, that's putting it kindly; the factory-driven extrusion process actually applies so much heat and pressure to the cereal grains that they liquefy. This slurry then allows the grains to be quickly and easily shaped into the flakes, puffs or other shapes that make the many distinct brands of cereal today so different.

Yet the calories in those original, relatively healthy flakes of corn, not being too far removed from the original ear of corn, equal the same number of calories you can find in the latter flakes (denatured as they are) – before, of course, the sugar spray adds a calorie or two more. Interestingly, as a devout Seventh Day Adventist, John Harvey refused to join the Kellogg's company because he thought that the addition of sugar lowered the health benefits of the cereal.

You can even consider making your own junk food. Admittedly, it's difficult to do at home, but a corn flake pelletizer or extrusion machine (with puffed extruder, also suitable for pet food) would set you back anything between £8,000 and £80,000 pounds depending on the quantities you wished to produce. According to one of the advertising brochures: '… nutritionally convenient food is produced by this process line, using grist as basic material, with different shapes such as granule, flake, animal, etc. One outstanding characteristic of the breakfast cereal is that it contains abundant compound carbohydrates and dietary fibre, strengthens lots of microelements, such as vitamins and minerals, and also can be added with cocoa and sugar, like honey and maltose'.

Or you could buy a:[150] '… traditional type Single & Double screw extruder machine using corn, rice or wheat flour as the raw material to produce snack food such as corn flakes, breakfast cereals, pet food, fish feed, etc. in various shapes by changing the mould'.

---

150 Extract from a well-known Chinese website selling manufacturing equipment, 2015.

191

To create your sludge first, you would need a powder mixing machine to mix your floury materials with water, emulsifiers and other additives. But to me, the funny thing is that according to the food labelling folks, what comes out at the end of this tortuous process has exactly the same protein, fat and carb contents – and even contains the same number of calories – as the fresh equivalent! To quote the tennis player John McEnroe, 'You have got to be joking!'. Where is the measure showing that fresh corn is better for you than the flavoured, extruded and dried version? Can such highly processed food really be as good for you as fresh produce? With my British understatement, I can safely say that I somewhat doubt that.

Some readers probably buy organic, fat-free cereal for the health reasons advertised on the box, but the fact is that the contents all just consist of extruded, highly refined carbs! The problem is not with the ingredients themselves, which are simple and seem 'whole' enough in the case of organic oats. The unhealthy aspect of boxed cereals is the violent processing required to manufacture them.

The manufacturing process used to make boxed cereal is so violent and denaturing that a proportion of the proteins in the grains are rendered toxic and allergenic as a result.[151] Because of the higher level of protein in the raw whole grains, this process leads to a breakfast cereal that's even more toxic than that found in cheap boxed cereals made with white flour. Such highly processed food would be better named denatured food, as far as I'm concerned.

You can look at this from different angles, but it's the refined carbs doing the damage, particularly when mixed with artificial emulsifiers that thicken the sludge and add shelf life. But we all know that processed foods are not just about cereals. You find them everywhere and sometimes you can carry out the comparative 'make it yourself' test. For example, a tasty home-made mayo contains eggs, olive oil, salt and maybe a little mustard. But in the UK, Tesco's Everyday Value Mayonnaise contains: Water, Rapeseed Oil (25%), Glucose-Fructose Syrup, Modified Maize Starch, Spirit Vinegar, Free Range Pasteurised Egg Yolk (2%), Salt,

151 Morell, 2005.

Acidity Regulator (Lactic Acid), Preservative (Sorbic Acid), Stabilisers (Xanthan Gum, Guar Gum) and Flavouring, which contains Mustard. These are also typical of the ingredients list, were you to see it, that go into a pre-prepared chicken mayo sandwich – plus, of course, the healthy wholemeal bread (Hovis wholemeal medium sliced bread, in this example) which contains: 64% Wholemeal Flour (Wheat), Water, Caramelised Sugar, Yeast, Soya Flour, Salt, Fermented Wheat Flour, Wheat Protein, Emulsifiers (E472e; E481), Vegetable Fat (Rapeseed; Palm) and Flour Treatment Agent (Ascorbic Acid).

In researching his book, *The Blue Zones: Lessons for Living Longer From the People Who've Lived the Longest*,[152] Dan Buettner travelled to long-lived communities around the world and tried to find common ground for their long and unusually healthy lives. Like Dr Wolf and his team of researchers back in Roseto, he returned stressing the importance of caring community values, but emphasised that diet and exercise (more in the natural sense of keeping active) were the other two factors, combined with a sense of purpose and spirituality.

In the island of Sardinia's long-lived upland hillside communities, Buettner speaks of meeting Thanasis and Eirini Karimalis, married in their early twenties and, at the time of writing, both in their late nineties. Their daily routine involved waking up naturally, working in the garden, having a late lunch and then following it up with a nap. Later, around sunset, they would visit neighbours and enjoy a glass of the local Cannonau wine; a wine, by the way, so rich in polyphenols as to have twice as much of them in one glass as there are in a whole bottle of Australian red (according to Roger Corder of the William Harvey Research Institute in London[153]). Their diet was also typical of others he met in the area: a breakfast of goats' milk, wine, sage tea or coffee, honey and flatbread ('pane carasau') made from local durum wheat. Lunch was almost always beans (lentils, garbanzos), potatoes, greens (fennel, dandelion or a spinach-like green called horta) and whatever seasonal vegetables their garden produced; dinner was bread and goats' milk. At

152 Buettner, 2008.
153 Smith, 2007.

Christmas and Easter, they would slaughter the family pig and enjoy small portions of larded pork for the next several months.

When we look at different communities and their diets around the world and compare them, I am often intrigued more by what they don't eat than by what they do. Sugar and tasty morsels like baked sweet pastries are only eaten as treats rather than as staples of their diet. Sugar is only used sparingly and high fructose corn syrup does not exist. Buettner reports that Dr Christina Chrysohoou, a cardiologist at the University of Athens, teamed up with half a dozen scientists to organize a study of Ikarians; Ikaria being a Greek island in the Aegean Sea. The study included a survey of the diet of 673 inhabitants. She found that her subjects consumed about six times as many beans each day as Americans, ate fish twice a week and meat five times a month, drank on average two to three cups of coffee a day and, importantly, took in about a quarter as much refined sugar. She also discovered that they were consuming high levels of olive oil along with two to four glasses of wine a day.[154]

The Western health model revolves around carb-loaded junk food, yet stresses the importance of exercise – while supporting a growing pharmaceutical industry and a huge market in vitamins and dietary supplements. Compare that with the fresh food diet and solid social structure which still thrives in Sardinia and on Ikaria; and used to thrive in the township of Roseto, Pennsylvania until the late 1960s.

---

154 Buettner, 2012.

One 'carb' film you need to see:
That Sugar Film

That Sugar Film is an Australian-made movie,[155] released in the UK in the summer of 2015. It sets out to inform us about what happens when we eat (and drink) too much sugar. Since sugar is added to around 80% of supermarket foods, it's difficult to avoid. But unlike in other recent films and documentaries on the subject that focus on the obvious suspects (sodas, cakes, desserts and the like), the film's star tries to eat a 'healthy' balanced diet. The film's actor-director, Damon Gameau, includes smoothies, low-fat yoghurts, cereals and granola bars in his sixty-day regime – but notably avoids soft drinks, confectionery and ice cream. So he's mixing in various slower-burning carbs like cereals and breads with the fructose and sucrose. 'I thought consuming a lot of foods like low-fat yoghurt and orange juice would be just fine,' he said in a New York Times article.[156] After all, he continued, 'these are the foods with flowers and bees and sunsets on their labels'. And that's what makes this film so different and so provocative. Coca-Cola, Snickers bars and doughnuts are typical of the usual culprits when we talk of 'the dangers' of excess sugar, but Damon avoided these completely. Yet surprisingly, he put on weight quickly. After just eighteen days, he had developed signs of fatty liver disease. And there were other noticeable effects. Despite continuing with his regular exercise routine, Damon gained 10cm of fat around his waist, developed mood swings and found it more and more difficult to exercise as the days passed. According to him, his daily calorie intake hadn't changed; he was simply dropping the avocados and nuts and other relatively high-calorie foods for low-fat produce and juices.

Most of us shake our heads when we hear that the average Western diet averages out to include between thirty and forty teaspoons of sugar a day, and our thoughts go first to sweet candies and maybe soft drinks.

---

155 2014.
156 O'Connor, 2015.

But the fact that these results came about when Damon Gameau was following the low-fat diet that we've all been prescribed for thirty-five years – that was a surprise. The hidden sugars in so-called healthy cereals, low-fat yoghurts and apple juice are hurting us more than we may think. That being said, Damon doesn't think that we should demonise just one nutrient. But noting again that sugar is now in 80% of all foods, he suggests sticking to the perimeter of the supermarket, where all the fresh foods are located. 'Buy real foods as much as you can' is now his motto. Unfortunately, the film is not that easy to view. However, at the time of writing, there is some good news for the UK: one group is looking to put the film into twelve thousand schools, and a full parliamentary screening of the film is scheduled.

More science? This book is intended for a broad reading public, and I am not a scientist. If you do want to read more on the subject, written at a more scientific level, try *The Art and Science of Low Carbohydrate Living*.[157] It was originally published for a medical audience, but most of it is accessible to the general public.

---

157 Volek et al., 2011.

Some surprising facts about our ancestors

One common line of thought goes simply that we are all living much longer today – so of course there is more diabetes and cancer (etc.) around. It's not that simple, though. High infant mortality levels in the past skewed the figures, making it look as if healthy adults had short lives. But they didn't. Taking a historical perspective, average life expectancy increased with age – once people had survived the higher mortality

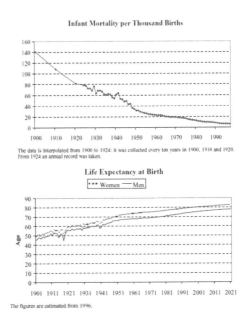

Infant Mortality per Thousand Births

The data is interpolated from 1900 to 1924: it was collected every ten years in 1900, 1910 and 1920. From 1924 an annual record was taken.

Life Expectancy at Birth

The figures are estimated from 1996.

Figure 19: These figures show the impact of improved children's health.

rates associated with childhood. So if we could take a trip back to when the Magna Carta was signed, exactly eight hundred years ago in medieval Britain, it might come as no surprise that life expectancy at birth would have been just thirty years. Consider this, however: if you had made it as far as being an adult and were a male member of the English aristocracy at the time, you could have expected to live to the ripe old age of 64 – a surprisingly long life, you might think. Medieval averages are listed here:[158]

- 1200–1300: to age 64;

- 1300–1400: to age 45 (the impact of the bubonic plague);

---

158 Lancaster, 1990, p.8.

- 1400–1500: to age 69;

- 1500–1550: to age 71.

It is a common myth that hundreds of years ago people used to die before they were forty or so. The facts show that if you made it to adulthood, you had a good chance of living a long life, even by today's standards. Infant mortality warps the average life expectancy statistics drastically; during the early 1600s in England, although two-thirds of all children died before the age of four, mature adult men lived on average to be seventy-one years of age.

Cause of Death in England and Wales: 1880 and 1997

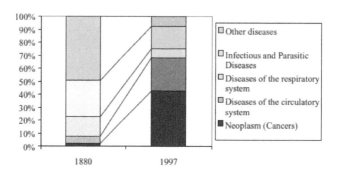

Figure 20:   Heart disease and cancer – the most common causes of death today.

This situation began to change around the year 1900. At this time, in the UK, around twenty-eight out of every two hundred children still died as infants. The 2005/2010 UN Statistics[159] show how this figure has now been driven down to just one in every two hundred children. Leading countries such as Sweden and Japan have reduced it to just one death in four hundred or even fewer. Stamping out child mortality is one of the greatest accomplishments of the twentieth century.

The other thing which has fundamentally changed relates to cause of death. Even taking into account the less reliable statistics from the end of the nineteenth century, very few people at that time died from cancer or circulatory system diseases (such as heart attacks). The figure for both

---

159 UNdata, 2012 revision.

causes combined in 1880 was below 10%, compared to 43% from cancer and a reported 26% from problems of the circulatory system in 1997.[160]

A study carried out in England and published in 2010[161] seems to support this line of thinking that to some extent, cancer is directly related to our lifestyle and diet. Lead researcher, Professor Rosalie David, of Manchester University's Faculty of Life Sciences commented in a press release that:[162] 'In industrialised societies, cancer is second only to cardiovascular disease as a cause of death. But in ancient times, it was extremely rare. There is nothing in the natural environment that can cause cancer. So it has to be a man-made disease, down to pollution and changes to our diet and lifestyle'.

Putting this all together, the main reason that life expectancy increased during the twentieth century is that we had become so effective at tackling infant mortality. And the main reason people died shifted from infectious and parasitic diseases to cancer and heart-related conditions. In the US, for example, in 2010, 53% of people died from cancer or heart disease. Interestingly, 6% of deaths were attributed to Alzheimer's and diabetes (and these percentages are rising fast).[163]

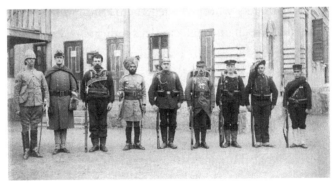

Figure 21:   Troops of the 1900 Eight Nations Alliance. Left to right: Britain, USA, Australia, India, Germany, France, Russia, Italy and Japan.

It may surprise you to read that paleo-pathologists have learned that the average human height has varied greatly over the centuries. But we

---

160 Crisp, 2010, p.48.
161 David and Zimmerman, 2010.
162 University of Manchester, 2010.
163 Blair Johnson et al., 2014.

have to go back to pre-farming times (at least ten thousand years) to gain a true perspective. Skeletons from Greek and Turkish hunter-gatherers from towards the end of the most recent ice age show that their average height was 5 feet 9 inches (1m 75cm) for men and 5 feet 5 inches (1m 64cm) for women; almost identical to their modern US counterparts. But this all changed as our antecedents turned to agricultural farming and quite literally set the seeds for today's population explosion. Average height crashed, and by 3000 BC had dropped to 5 feet 3 inches (1m 60cm) for men and 5 feet (just over 1m 50cm) for women. By classical times, heights were very slowly on the rise again – but modern Greeks and Turks have still not quite regained the average height of their distant ancestors.[164]

The anthropologist Jared Diamond has explored the health of those early farmers as they emerged from their previous hunter-gatherer communities, and he refers to the excavation of some eight hundred skeletons in modern day Illinois.[165] This paints a picture of the health changes that occurred when, at that location in around AD 1150, a hunter-gatherer culture gave way to intensive maize farming. Compared to the hunter-gatherers who preceded them, the farmers had a nearly 50% increase in bone enamel defects. This indicates severe malnutrition, together with other diseases; in particular, an increase in degenerative conditions of the spine – possibly due to their hard physical labour in the fields.

Earlier hunter-gatherer communities subsisted mostly by foraging. Dating back nearly two million years, they have enjoyed the longest-lasting lifestyle that humans have experienced to date. Some ten thousand years ago, they were faced with a choice: whether to continue limiting population growth through food scarcity or to try to increase food production. They chose the latter. What we have as a result today is the efficient mass farming of animals and particularly of cereal crops. This has allowed us to grow to a global population of over seven billion.

164 Diamond, 1987. (Quote in text box is from the same source.)
165 Idem.

In contrast to those earlier hunter-gatherers, who enjoyed a varied diet, the first farmers and farm workers got much of their food from a very limited number of starchy grass crops. The process of reducing the biodiversity of our guts started at that point. These cheaper, more accessible calories came at the cost of poor nutrition – although, even today, we don't seem to have fully accepted that. In

'Forced to choose between limiting population or trying to increase food production, we chose the latter and ended up with starvation, warfare, and tyranny.'

Source: Jared Diamond, the Pulitzer Prize-winning author and anthropologist.

my opinion, it's high time we faced up to it. Today, the triumvirate of wheat, rice and maize, which provides 60% of the world's energy intake, provides the bulk of what we human beings eat. Yet each of the three brings with it questionable nutritional benefits and problems; particularly in the highly processed and modified forms we seem to prefer. Although the domestication of all three major forms of carbohydrate began ten thousand or so years ago, the expansion of agriculture was slow; it impacted countries and local communities at different times. Rice, for example, experienced its major expansion from Central China into India just four thousand years ago.[166]

Roots and tubers still make up a large part of the diet in parts of Africa, where hunter-gatherer diets live on to a certain extent. But with Westernised diets moving in, this is destined to change. Since 1970, consumption of roots and tubers in the Pacific Islands has fallen by 8%. Cereal consumption has jumped by 40%, from 61 to 85 kilograms per person per year.[167] It should be no surprise that they lead the world in terms of obesity and type-2 diabetes.[168]

---

166 Harris (ed.), 1996.
167 Forbes Magazine, 2007.
168 International Diabetes Federation, 2013.

Evolving bigger brains by learning to cook food

Eating salad and a certain proportion of raw vegetables is good for us, but too much of them can lead to an upset stomach. For a long time now, we have been able to draw more nutrients from cooked food than from raw. The latest evidence is that cooking foods began nearly two million years ago, a lot earlier than previously thought. Richard Wrangham, Professor of Biological Anthropology at Harvard University believes that learning to cook with fire spurred on the development of modern humans. 'I cook, therefore I am' is his mantra. 'I tend to think of the advent of cooking as having a huge impact on the quality of the diet,' he says.[169] 'In fact, I can't think of any increase in the quality of diet in the history of life that is bigger. And repeatedly we have evidence in biology of increases in dietary quality affecting bodies. The food was softer, easier to eat, with a higher density of calories – so this led to smaller guts, and, since the food was providing more energy, we see more evidence of energy use by the body. There's only one time it could have happened on that basis; that is, with the evolution of *Homo erectus* somewhere between 1.6 and 1.8 million years ago.'

When we take a look at our ancestors, *Homo erectus* is the species demonstrating the biggest drop in tooth size in human evolution. Our ancestors' ribs used to point out in a similar way to those of chimpanzees and gorillas, to make room for their big bellies and large digestive systems. But that all changed with our cooked food and reduced digestive needs; the ribs flattened as we stood tall, and, at the same time, our brains grew further in size.

Cooking meant that we no longer needed large teeth for cutting and chewing food, and the resulting smaller guts stimulated blood flow to our growing and bigger brains. Going back to the popular bumper

---

169 Wrangham, 2009, Chapter: *Introduction.*

sticker 'I cook, therefore I am', it may be better expressed as 'I cook, therefore my teeth and stomach are smaller, but my brain is bigger'.

What are carbohydrates, and do they add to a healthy diet?

Carbohydrates are the main constituents in those allegedly harmless comfort foods (such as bread, potatoes and rice) that fill us up. We've been brought up learning that fat is bad and that protein is good – but when combined together with the supposedly innocuous 'carbs', they form the triumvirate that rules our lives. We eat them every day – unless we are fasting – and the proportions and quantities of these macro-nutrients (as the nutritionists call them) determine whether we put on weight, the amount of energy we dispose of and whether our vital organs will function correctly. A balanced diet, we are told, is a healthy diet that will bring us to a ripe old age before even those gifted with the strongest genes begin to fade into that third age that precedes death.

That's all very cheerful, you might be thinking – but what constitutes a balanced and healthy diet is hotly contested among the so-called experts. And even the relative value of these three key uber-nutrients is now in doubt. Yes, doctors and dieticians seem pretty happy to say that a certain amount of protein is necessary, but when it comes to fat, they're all over the place. As for carbohydrates (that's basically starches and sugars), their role is now seriously being questioned by a significant minority of doctors and researchers. The thing is, they are less innocuous than we have been led to believe. Carbs do more to spike your essential hormonal activities (such as insulin) than either fats or proteins do. As you have r hormonal activity drives so much of how our body uses food to put on fat and add muscle, but it also helps indicate when you feel full. If that circuitry is disrupted, it affects the whole body and can lead to poor health – and, of course, to putting on the pounds.

Go into your average coffee bar, be it mainstream like Costa or Starbucks or artisanal like my favourite (Monmouth Coffee House in Covent Garden), and you also will be presented with pastries, buns and scones featuring two main ingredients: sugar and flour. The carbs get us twice because both the sugar and the flour join forces with fat and protein to make the saliva-inducing mixture that we crave. Finding something low in carbs at these counters is nigh on impossible, with a typical Blueberry Muffin (Starbucks) checking in at 50% of the calorific value as carbs – a full 28% of the total taking the form of sugar.

It's just the same with industrially made snack bars. People have attacked their high fat levels, but the reality is that a Snickers bar, for example, contains 63% carbohydrate content by weight. Nearly half of the bar is pure sugar – 47%, to be precise.

Of the three main types of carbohydrate we eat (starches, sugars and fibre), fibre will be only partly digested; most passes through your body. But starches and sugars follow other journeys. Starches, or complex carbohydrates, consist of long chains of sugar molecules known more correctly as polysaccharides and oligosaccharides. You find them in plant-based foods like potatoes, rice and grains and your digestive tract breaks down these long sugar chains into single sugars. In effect, this means that your body treats all carbs as sugar; what differs is that some carbs are digested and turned into sugar more slowly (that's what the Glycaemic Index refers to). The chemical name of white table sugar is sucrose – a 50/50 mix of glucose and fructose. But whereas glucose is rapidly absorbed into the bloodstream, fructose goes directly to the liver, where it is converted to glycogen. For lack of storage space, excess fructose will be turned into body fat.

Sugar (in its powdery form or when found naturally in milk, fruit and sweet-tasting syrups such as maple and honey) provides you with a short-term energy boost – but once you start eating, it is highly addictive. Try eating one chocolate from a box and leaving the rest for another day. Most of us struggle to do that.

Now, the official line is that the type of carbohydrate you choose to eat matters because some sources are healthier than others. Dieticians love to tout the benefit of 'healthy, whole-grain' breads made from whole wheat, rye, barley and quinoa. They usually advise that these represent better choices than refined white bread or French fries. But to your body there's not a lot of difference. The carbs that you eat will all be digested and processed as sugar, following a pathway that's similar to (if somewhat slower than) what would happen if you were eating sweets. The apparently healthy whole-wheat thing has a lot to do with how fibre has been marketed over the years. Visually, it just looks as if it's more fibrous – but looks have little to do with true fibre content. Some bread manufacturers simply add colouring to deepen the shade of brown, but looks can deceive in other ways. Back in 2007, research results were published showing that fresh coffee contains up to ¾ of a gram of fibre per 100 millilitres, even though you cannot see it. Consuming a cup of coffee – say a 'grande' (medium-sized) cup at Starbucks – will fill you with around 3 grams of fibre. This is roughly the same as a raw apple and 20% or more of the average American's recommended daily intake.

Many people get confused about carbohydrates, but you'll find them in all vegetables, to some extent. Lowering your intake means focusing on certain foods, especially those veggies that grow above the ground (such as courgettes, beans and peas), before steadily adding in carrots, onions and other root vegetables at a later stage. Potatoes have to be eaten as a small accompaniment or left for special occasions, I'm afraid!

Carbohydrates provide the body (and in particular, the brain) with glucose, but if you look back to our ancestors of the past couple of million years, regular access to carbs was limited. This is presumably why the body has an alternative supply to the brain – it starts to produce ketones as a replacement fuel for your brain when carbs are in short supply. (This was covered in more detail in 'Going ketogenic' on page 112.)

Oils and fats

Generally, we call something a fat if it's solid at room temperature and an oil if it's in a liquid form. Chemically, they are the same, although saturated fats tend to be more stable and hence solid. That's why, depending on your kitchen's temperature, coconut oil (which melts at about 24°C) may be seen as a fat or an oil – it's your choice to name. Whether an oil is resistant to oxidisation and going rancid at either high or low heat depends on the relative degree of saturation of the fatty acids in it. Both saturated and mono-unsaturated fats are resistant to heat, reducing the chance of oxidisation; that provided another reason why, in Katy's diet, we cut back on the use of poly-unsaturated fats such as corn and sunflower oil, using them only in small quantities together with olive oil in mayonnaise and salad dressing.

Olive oil deserves an early mention, since it's a so-called essential part of the much-touted Mediterranean diet – even though its use in cooking was limited in the past. Olive oil is a relatively stable mono-unsaturated fat. It also contains 12-14% saturated fat, so it keeps well. It's still advisable to store olive oil in a dark place or at least in a can or a dark bottle to stop any oxidisation. Interestingly, some nutritionists warn against it because of the saturated fat that it contains – I would argue that this is beneficial.

What about margarine, which is a form of chemically thickened vegetable oil? Following a period when the world fell in love with margarine and told us that saturated fats like butter, lard and coconut oil were bad for our hearts, there is now growing evidence that saturated fats and oils are, in fact, better for us. According to Marcia Otto (Assistant Professor of Epidemiology at the University of Texas), by warning people against full-fat dairy foods, the United States is 'losing a huge opportunity for the prevention of disease'.[170] As the lead author of large studies

---

170 As reported by Whoriskey, 2015 (2).

published in 2012[171] and 2013[172] which were funded by government and academic institutions rather than the industry, she continues: 'What we have learned over the last decade is that certain foods that are high in fat seem to be beneficial'.

Research from Canada's McMaster University has found that saturated fats are not associated with an increased risk of death, heart disease, stroke or type-2 diabetes.[173] The publication of this research was followed up by a number of opinion pieces, including comments from Dr Hassan Chamsi-Pasha of the King Fahd Armed Forces Hospital in Jeddah, Saudi Arabia. He wrote that:[174] 'Five decades of controversy surrounding basic dietary guidelines and nutrition recommendations is a public acknowledgement of a failed research paradigm'.

Yet to date, government guidelines around the world still tell us to make low-fat choices, even though no-one disputes that the eating of fat facilitates important biochemical processes in our digestive systems. Dietary fat, which is also a constituent of many of the foods you eat, is crucial to the absorption of the fat-soluble vitamins – particularly vitamins A, D, K and E. It is the ability of these vitamins to dissolve in fat that allows for that absorption. This occurs through their movement across the cell walls of the small intestine and into the body's general circulation. The vitamins progress through the intestine, into the bloodstream and then to the liver, where they are stored until the body needs them. Without enough fat in your diet, your body is unable to effectively absorb these essential fat-soluble vitamins.

Three degrees of saturation

OK – here's the technical bit: there's saturated fat, mono-unsaturated fat and poly-unsaturated fat; the first two being more resistant to heating.

Of these, there are two main types of poly-unsaturated fat. These are known as omega-3 fatty acids and omega-6 fatty acids ('essential'

---

171 Otto et al., 2012.
172 Otto et al., 2013.
173 de Souza et al., 2015.
174 Chamsi-Passa, 2015.

fatty acids), which the body needs because it cannot make them itself. Generally, doctors agree that our diets have become too rich in omega-6, so we need to seek out as many ways of ingesting omega-3 as possible – preferably through eating more fresh foods (like oily fish) rather than through taking supplements in the form of pills. On this message, all nutritionists agree – though many advocate supplements in the form of fish-oil pills and the like, which I have come to believe are not the best solution.

In fact, what the most recent research is telling us is that it's even more important to reduce the amount of 'inflammatory' omega-6 that we take in (mostly in the form of seed oils such as corn, safflower, soy, sunflower, etc.) than it is to increase omega-3 intake.

Italians know best: The Colonnata Lard Festival

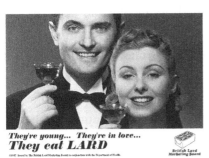

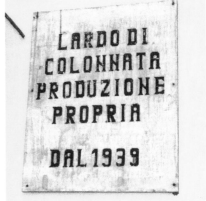

Figure 22: Yes – there really did used to be a British Lard Marketing Board. This ad is from 1958.

Figure 23: Shop sign; photo taken at the Colonatta Lard Festival, every August in Tuscany.

After years of propaganda, many of us have effectively been brainwashed into believing the evils of saturated fat. Nothing visually represents our thoughts more than a piece of lard – usually rendered pork fat. This is kind of funny because in fact, lard contains more mono-unsaturated than saturated fat. But in places like Italy, where lard is still used extensively in making pastry as well as in stove top cooking, the tradition of producing lard has been passed down from generation to generation. Today, there are only a few families in Colonnata, Tuscany who are full-time producers of artisanal lard. But every year, in August, the 'Festival of the Lard' is held there. If you were to find yourself in Tuscany at that time of year, it would present the best opportunity to taste their delicious organic lard in a variety of dishes. In terms of nutrition, we should also note that lard contains about half the level of saturated fat as coconut oil (or palm kernel oil, for that matter) and that its 40% saturated fat level is lower than the level found in butter, which averages out at between 50 and 60% depending on the quality. Remember olive oil, everyone's 'go to' oil today, also contains saturated fat – usually coming in at between 12 and 14%. But there again, if saturated fat is good for us (as it may well be) … why be defensive about it?

A little oily history

The crushing of olives and reported use of olive oil goes back to before the birth of Christ, although usage back then was primarily for heating and lighting – and, in ancient Greek times, as a body rub used particularly for adorning athletes. Zoom forward to 1830, and sunflower seeds were first being crushed in Western Russia to produce commercial quantities of oil for use as animal fodder, for cosmetic purposes and for human consumption. The very first production of corn oil took place in the USA in 1889, and commercial soybean oil dates from the 1930s. It's interesting to note that those vegetable oils that we consume in large quantities today are manufactured by an industry that was still in its infancy just over a hundred years ago. It goes without saying that it is much cheaper for manufacturers to make food with oils chemically extracted from plant seeds than it is to raise animals for their fat … and this dovetails nicely into the conventional wisdom that reducing heart disease means prioritising these unsaturated vegetable oils over saturated animal fats. Prepared and processed foods are often labelled as containing vegetable oils, without any further explanatory details; you'll find them in potato chips, sweets and candies, frozen foods, canned soups and most prepared meals.

To process these edible vegetable oils, water in the form of steam bubbles up through the oil, removing water-soluble chemicals and other impurities that can leave unwanted flavours and smells. This, together with a further chemical deodorisation process, also lightens the colour of the oil.

Although these oils are labelled as 'vegetable' oils, when you think about it, excepting olive oil, vegetable oil does not really exist! Veggies aren't very oily. Fruit oils such as coconut, palm and even avocado do exist – as do nut oils like macadamia, peanut and pecan. But it is seed oils like canola, sunflower, safflower, maize, soybean, cottonseed, grapeseed, rice bran, etc. which make up the industrial mainstream. While fruit and nut oils can be beneficial, seed oils are nowadays considered by a growing minority to pose a health risk, particularly when heated. Yet you cannot buy packaged or takeaway food that is cooked in anything but seed oil, and these prepared dishes all contain high and potentially damaging levels of omega-6 fatty acids.

Potato chips (crisps) are a typical example of how we take in large quantities of seed oil in the processed foods we eat. Kettle Chips, for example, contain about 30% by weight of sunflower, safflower or corn oil – depending upon the country in which you buy them. Potato is still the dominant ingredient, with just under 60% of the weight. But for reference, a recent ingredient list shows the following: potatoes, safflower and/or sunflower and/or canola oil, maltodextrin, sea salt, salt, green bell pepper powder, garlic powder, sugar, yeast extract, spices, vinegar, jalapeno powder, onion powder, parsley powder, citric acid, natural flavours and parsley flakes. All the more reason to start making your own crispy wafers of potato, parsnip, beetroot and other vegetables?

A growing number of holistic doctors and researchers[175] suggest that we should strive for a 1:1 ratio between these two types of essential fatty acid – but with our typical Western diet, that ain't easy! Our typical

---

175 See Simopoulos, 2002.

intake ratio of omega-6 to omega-3 is something between 5:1 and 10:1 or more, which leads to high levels of omega-6 and residual inflammation within your body – both bad for your general health and associated with heart disease, cancer and … and … so, where is all our omega-6 coming from today?

Go back fifty or a hundred years and most of the fat in our diet was of the grass-fed animal variety or from nuts and fish. As you will read in more detail later, the meat and dairy produce from grass-fed cattle contains much higher levels of omega-3. What we eat is very different today. In today's processed, packaged and pre-prepared food, sunflower, corn, soy and safflower seed oils are commonly used, containing an omega-6 content of up to 75%. This exacerbates the inflammation in your body (referred to earlier – page 31) and puts you at risk of disease. For example, McDonald's restaurants use a blend of seven ingredients in their frying oil, including: canola oil, corn oil, soybean oil and hydrogenated soybean oil with tert-Butylhydroquinone (TBHQ), citric acid and dimethylpolysiloxane. The funny thing is, they used to use beef tallow until the 1980s, when saturated fats got a bad name!

Oil	Omega-6 Content	Omega-3 Content
Safflower	75%	0%
Sunflower	65%	0%
Corn	54%	0%
Cottonseed	50%	0%
Sesame	42%	0%
Peanut	32%	0%
Soybean	51%	7%
Canola	20%	9%
Walnut	52%	10%
Olive	9%	1%
Flaxseed	14%	57%
Fish	0%	100%

Figure 24: Omega-6 vs Omega-3 content in oils.

But what are the alternatives? Hemp seed oil, cold-pressed flax oil and walnut oil are high in omega-3. These taste great on salads, but they are essentially unstable, just like avocado and macadamia nut oils (which are also good, if expensive). Like most oils, they have a relatively short shelf life and need to be kept in dark cabinets away from oxygen and light to stop them going rancid. Best of all, keep them in the fridge in dark glass bottles! Just drizzle them on your favourite salad or veggies for flavour and then put them away. That doesn't really help with frying, though, does it? (Yes, you guessed it – they are heat-sensitive too, and, excepting macadamia nut oil, have lower burn points!) Coconut oil, lard from free-range pigs, purified butter or ghee are better cooking options. They are more stable and suitable for higher temperatures.

So stop using vegetable oils like sunflower oil, safflower oil, soybean and corn oil, which are all high in omega-6 acids. That's also another reason to avoid pre-packaged, processed foods as much as possible. To dial up the omega-3, increase your intake of fatty fish such as salmon, tuna, mackerel, anchovies and sardines. These fish are all sources of omega-3 fatty acids, and you benefit by decreasing the level of inflammation in your body. As you'll have read, nutritionists and dieticians disagree on many things, but there is unanimity about this. Increase the proportion of omega-3 to omega-6 fats that you eat; this will be beneficial for your health and help your body in an anti-inflammatory way.

The top ten sources of omega-3 fats you can include in your diet are:

- Flax seeds (also known as linseed);

- Walnuts;

- Sardines;

- Salmon;

- Brussels sprouts;

- Cauliflower;

- Mustard seeds;

- Soybeans/Tofu
  (though some are concerned with the GM content);

- Shrimp;

- Broccoli.

The omega-3 you eat in the form of meat, eggs and fish is easier for the body to assimilate. When it comes to meat, omega-3 and 6 levels vary according to the animal's diet. For cattle, regardless of whether your beef is grain-fed or grass-fed, you'll be getting about 40-50% saturated fat, about 40-50% mono-unsaturated fat and somewhere near 10% poly-unsaturated fat. The most current research indicates that beef contains consistent levels of omega-6, regardless of diet. That's good news if you can't afford grass-fed beef. At least grain-fed beef won't be adding much to the already high levels of omega-6 that you're probably eating every day. But significantly higher levels of omega-3 are still to be found in grass-fed beef. So, why not try grass-fed beef and economise with a slightly smaller portion size or a cheaper cut? Or try cooking offal, which is particularly rich in many vitamins and minerals. Sheep and goats are mostly raised free-range, so you're safe there. The same general rule goes for free-range pork such as Black Iberian and for free-range chickens too.

The ignored 1960s US military test – eight years in the making

The anti-fat movement became so strong in the second half of the twentieth century that even conclusive research results were set aside if they didn't fit the mould. One of the largest human trials examining the effects of replacing animal fats with seed oils was known as the Los Angeles Veterans Trial, completed way back in 1969.[176] It was conducted with 846 Californian military veterans, who were randomly assigned to two different hostel kitchens. One kitchen replaced all animal-fat products with corn oil for the eight-year duration of the study. The other kitchen kept on with its normal high-animal-fat diet.

The purpose of the trial was to determine what heart disease-related benefits were linked to removing animal fats from the diet. The thing was … there were none. The seed-oil group had a slightly lower average blood-cholesterol level, but heart disease-related events were not significantly different between the two groups (in keeping with what we now know of the lack of connection between levels of cholesterol

---

176 Dayton et al., 1969.

and heart disease). Yet there was a different, wholly unexpected result: a dramatic difference in cancer deaths between the two groups. After eight years, the incidence of fatal cancers in the seed-oil group nearly doubled that of the normal-diet group. It may be old research, but it does provide a further reminder of how we should be eating today.

Oxidised cholesterol – the real culprit in heart disease

Dr Fred Kummerow (see Kummerow, 2013) analysed the arteries and blood of patients who had undergone heart bypass operations. He found elevated levels of oxidised cholesterols, called oxysterols. 'These cholesterol derivatives are the real culprit in the development of heart disease,' Kummerow said in a 2013 interview with futuremedicine.com, '… and frying foods in overused oil or smoking cigarettes can oxidise cholesterol, creating these derivatives.'

His work in the 1970s was largely ignored at the time. More at the www. fatisourfriend.com blog,

---

So, which fat is your best friend?

It depends! There's a lot of information out there, some of it conflicting. A number of the different so-called experts have quite different things to say. So, on balance, these are the considered opinions of this writer (after a lot of reading and talking to people in the health and nutrition business). You can find much more on the subject at the website: www.fatisourfriend.com. What is important to know is that the food scientists and nutritionists who scared us away from cooking with saturated fats got things wrong. Your great-grandmother may have cooked with lard, goose fat, butter, ghee, palm or coconut oil, depending upon which part of the world she grew up in, but she knew best.

Which fat for frying?

Don't use the typically large bottles of cheap vegetable and seed oil such as sunflower and corn oil. They contain too high a proportion of omega-6 fatty acids, which most of us get too much of in our diets; in addition, some of the commercial processing methods are questionable. Being poly-unsaturated, they are also inherently unstable – they give off dangerous chemicals when heated for frying and go rancid much quicker than other oils. The 'least bad' of these big-bottle solutions is probably rapeseed oil (sometimes marketed as colza). Remember, though, that it is highly processed, purified and bleached before it passes through a deodoriser to take away the 'cabbagy' smell – although, to its advantage, it is richer in omega-3.

I believe that saturated fats are good for you, so it's OK (even beneficial to your health) to use beef dripping, lard and goose fat! Coconut oil, another saturated fat which is sometimes labelled coconut butter, is heart-healthy – as is organic palm oil. They don't go rancid, and they have a high smoke point, so they are great for frying. Some people say they impart too much taste, but (particularly with coconut oil) it's mostly the smell which sometimes reminds you of its origins.

The cheaper olive oils have a higher smoke point too, but they go rancid more quickly than the above-mentioned fats and oils, so make sure that you store them in a cool, dark place.

Ghee tastes good, and you can easily make your own (or other forms of clarified butter, all being safer at higher cooking temperatures). Store them (for months, if needed) in your fridge; ghee adds great taste and resists oxidisation.

Which oil for salads?

Home-made 'mayo' tastes delicious. It's healthier than store-bought because you know exactly what goes into it and there is no need to add preservatives. It will keep for up to a week in the fridge. My favourite mixtures include using a 50:50 blend of extra-virgin olive oil and cold-pressed organic rapeseed as the base. Salads dressed with olive oil and a dash of a stronger-flavoured nut oil are also delicious. Use cold-pressed, organic versions when possible; quantities can be small and so won't hit the wallet too hard. This ensures they are as fresh as possible before being stored – as with all oils – in a cool, dark place.

For more flavour in a salad, add a little of any nut oils (such as walnut, macadamia, almond or hazelnut) to taste, or make your own herb infusions. Basil- and chive-flavoured olive oil are particularly delicious.

Summary – When you are cooking and frying

Lard and beef dripping (tallow): these are stable fats that do not easily go rancid and that allow for cooking at higher temperatures. Grass-fed animals, if you can find them, result in fats with higher levels of omega-3.

Duck and goose fat: these are splendid on roast potatoes (limit your quantity), according to Gordon Ramsay, with a long shelf life and vitamin-absorbing benefits.

Coconut: this healthy, largely saturated oil is semi-solid at room temperature and lasts for months without going rancid. Try to choose virgin coconut oil. It's organic, tastes good and has associated health benefits.

Palm oil: a tricky one, this – palm oil is derived from the fruit of oil palms, making it a good choice for all forms of cooking. Unrefined red palm oil is best, but there are concerns about the sustainability of harvesting palm oil, as growing the trees means less free space for indigenous animal populations.

Butter: this was demonised in the past due to its high saturated fat content, but it really is healthy and nutritious. It contains vitamins A, E and K2, and is rich in particular fatty acids which have been shown to lower body fat percentage in humans, fight inflammation and improve gut health. It's best to keep it covered to stop the oxidisation, which discolours the surface after a while. You often buy it ready-salted now, but salted butter was actually developed to prevent spoilage and mask the rancid taste that can develop over time; this is not unhealthy, but is certainly less pleasing to the taste buds!

Ghee: melting butter gently and separating the non-fat element makes it more suitable for cooking. The resulting ghee is a staple of much Indian cuisine. It has a usefully high smoke point of 250°C.

Olive oil: for preference, use first-pressed extra-virgin olive oil. The manufacturing process is less industrial, it tastes better, and it contains more nutrients and antioxidants than the refined variety. That being said, if you like to fry food in a deep fryer from time to time, it makes sense to buy the cheaper non-virgin variety. It can go rancid, though, so keep olive oil in a cool, dry, dark place.

Fish oil: … by the way, is a great source of omega-3 fatty acids. However, it is generally only used as a supplement. Eating oily fish such as sardines, mackerel and salmon is considered to be heart-healthy – one other thing that all nutritionists agree upon!

Summary – For salads: dressing, drizzling and mayonnaise

Flax oil: this contains lots of the plant form of omega-3, which is good for us. But the human body doesn't easily convert this vegetable form of omega-3 into the most active forms (which the body is able digest). It is not really suitable for cooking.

Olive oil: reappearing on this list; use the best and tastiest cold-pressed extra-virgin variety you can afford.

Nut oils: there are many nut oils available, most of which are used for flavouring – in salads, for example. Because they are rich in poly-unsaturated fats, they are not the best choice for cooking; they oxidise easily. Peanuts (which are actually 'legumes', not nuts) have a similar composition, so the oil is also liable to oxidise at high heat. There is one nutty exception, which is macadamia nut oil; it contains mostly mono-unsaturated fats (just like olive oil), but in most countries it is expensive and quite difficult to find.

A further word about seed and vegetable oils: I know – this is the difficult bit; we've heard for years that these are generally better for us than lard and butter etc. But they are not. They are made in huge quantities in industrial processing plants and are very rich in omega-6 fatty acids. Not only should you not cook with them, you should probably avoid them altogether – not that avoidance is really an option. They are ubiquitous in most processed foods, and are used for 'heart-healthy' reasons by many chefs! They have been praised by the media and many nutrition professionals since the 1970s, but an increasing amount of research is beginning to link the use of these oils with heart disease and auto-immune diseases such as cancer – particularly when you fry at higher temperatures with them.

Avoid them, that is, unless you find artisanal versions and choose to use them as an occasional salad dressing. They include: sunflower, sesame, soybean, corn, cottonseed, canola (not widely sold in Europe), rapeseed (admittedly higher in omega-3 – but still industrialised production), grapeseed, safflower and rice bran oils. One associated problem with eating too many pre-prepared, processed and packaged meals is that they invariably contain 'some of the above' oils in surprisingly large quantities. Potato crisps lead the way with around 30% sunflower oil as the norm in Europe.

Why full-fat 'regular' milk is best

Once a week, my niece Ellie buys in what she calls 'normal milk' (i.e. 2% fat) to stock her grandmother's fridge so that when tea or coffee is served to visitors, they can get the 2% milk they are used to. She doesn't think it's right to force Grandma's guests to add what she calls 'fatty milk' to their cups of tea. Here, she is of course referring to the 4% full-fat version, which older generations in their turn still call 'normal milk'. I should mention that Ellie's grandmother has been drinking 'normal milk' for all of her eighty-seven years.

How times have changed. In fact, when was the last time you heard someone ask for 'Full-fat milk, please,' at Starbucks or Costa? 'Is it low-fat milk?' or 'Skimmed milk, please,' are more frequently heard. Then, of course, there are the soy milk advocates. This is much-needed for those with genuine milk allergies, yet is also in demand for a growing clique who consider their blended and strained soy bean extract to be contributing to their wellbeing.

'What's wrong with that?' I hear you say. Everyone knows that animal fats are bad for us. Even the UK Dairy Council informs us that: 'full-fat milk contains saturated fats which raise cholesterol which in turn increases your risk of cardiovascular disease (CVD, or, for the layman, heart attacks and strokes)'. On their website, they further advise us to:[177] '… eat a diet containing fruit, vegetables and wholegrain, with moderate intakes of legumes, nuts and **low-fat dairy** …'.

Yet recent studies contradict this 'fact' – or, should I say, this negative assumption about drinking full milk or eating real butter. A good review of the subject matter appeared in the March 5th 2015 issue of *Time* magazine.[178] The research shows that there are great benefits to consuming full-fat milk and dairy products; they actually help prevent obesity, diabetes and even (ironically) cardiovascular disease itself. Now,

---

177 The Dairy Council, n.d.
178 Heid, 2015.

the UK Dairy Council is, of course, government-funded, so it probably has no choice but to pay heed to today's official health warnings.

These days, so called conventional wisdom gets us automatically associating full-fat products such as milk, cheese and butter with future illness and weight gain. The fact that our grandparents and their ancestors found it perfectly normal to eat these natural products holds little or no sway. In today's mythology, we assume that they probably died younger because of their dietary mistakes. Yet in fact as we learned, although infant mortality rates have declined and today's medicines can add a couple of years to our lives in old age, we're not really living longer – in spite of our 'healthy' diets. If anything, low-fat products are contributing to a growing number of diseases; namely diabetes, cancer and Alzheimer's. So, dear reader: how does it feel to have been effectively brainwashed? Because you almost certainly, instinctively, feel that full-fat milk and cheese is bad for your health.

Just yesterday, I was sitting with my other sister-in-law, Tricia as she took a delicious piece of sourdough bread spread with local farmyard butter and described it as a 'naughty pleasure'. Was she thinking of the high level of carbohydrates and opiate-like chemicals found in wheat flour – or was the naughty pleasure to be found in the consumption of butter? No discussion: it was, of course, the butter.

Tricia was participating in the quasi-religious delight we experience in Western societies, associated with the concept of 'sinning'. When it comes to food, it's based on the false premise that if something tastes good, it must be bad for you. Yet do you really think that eating tasteless, reduced-fat cheese and 'healthier' butter that's been mixed with treated seed oils or drinking bland-tasting skimmed milk is how God meant things to be (I'm only guessing here!)? Surely, if so, (S)He would have provided cows with two types of udder – one to squeeze out the skimmed milk and the other (just for special occasions) for the fresh cream.

There is now an increasing amount of evidence which shows that if you opt for low-fat versions of dairy products, you are more likely to become obese than are those weird folks who eat the dairy products in their unadulterated, full-fat form. Yet school districts across the United

States have banned whole milk, serving low-fat or no-fat options instead (Bill Clinton's well-intentioned foundation has been a major player in this effort). School kids in the US have been found to drink greater quantities of the low-fat milk, which is what they mostly receive these days, because there is a lesser feeling of satiety that goes with it. They simply never feel really full, so they drink more.

A recent meta-analysis of sixteen relevant studies published in the *European Journal of Nutrition*[179] showed that **consumption of full-fat dairy products is correlated with a lower risk of gaining weight.** But higher-fat milk has more calories. How can this be? Part of the reason, again, is that you simply feel fuller after smaller quantities of real food. Here are a few factoids about drinking regular full-fat milk:

- Scientific analyses of some of the compounds found in high-fat dairy products have shown that they have beneficial effects on the colon and that they reduce inflammation in the gastrointestinal tract.

- Full-fat dairy has been shown to reduce the level of triglycerides in your blood and improve insulin sensitivity.

- Dairy fat is a good source of fat-soluble vitamins like retinol (active vitamin A) and vitamin K2, which are difficult to obtain elsewhere in the diet.

Other research is also supportive. The headline in *Science Daily* on April 2nd 2015 read:[180] 'Consumption of high-fat dairy products associated with a lower risk of developing diabetes'. A 2009 Swedish study of 1,732 rural men in the *International Journal of Environmental Research and Public Health*[181] found that eating fruits and vegetables didn't lower the risk of coronary heart disease ... **unless they were consumed together with high-fat dairy products!** To be precise: 'Daily intake of fruit and vegetables was associated with a lower risk of coronary heart

---

179 Kratz et al., 2013.
180 Lund University, 2015.
181 Holmberg et al., 2009.

disease when combined with a high dairy fat consumption but not when combined with a low dairy fat consumption. Choosing wholemeal bread or eating fish at least twice a week showed no association with the outcome'.

The results shouldn't surprise us, but somehow they still do. Many of the vitamins and micronutrients in food are fat-soluble, which means they cannot be absorbed without the presence of adequate fat. Put differently: if you eat fruits or vegetables without fat, you'll absorb only a fraction of the nutrients you would absorb if you ate them with fat. The question seems to be coming round to: how much are we risking our health with the current low-fat food fad? The processed food manufacturers love it; after removing the fat, they have to replace it with something tasty or be able to thicken food differently. They do this by using sugar, salt and various starchy, inexpensive carbs. Of course, a myriad of chemicals and gums are also added to enhance the eating experience.

So, this is the way my anti-brainwashing mantra is heading: I suggest that when it comes to dairy, following these simple rules will make you feel fuller. So please, again – don't count the calories:

- Use real, full-fat milk in your coffee or add some cream made from grass-fed cows.

- Eat full-fat yoghurt made from whole milk – it tastes better and is better for you.

- Skip the 'fake' spreads made with vegetable oils – choose butter.

- Cook with butter (as well as, not instead of, lard and coconut oil), clarified butter or ghee. The last two are both inherently stable, don't oxidise and have a higher burn point (and are easy to make at home).

- Select the tasty, high-fat cheeses that you like best.

- If you've got kids and they don't enjoy veggies, melt some butter and dip their veggies – you'll be surprised how popular broccoli becomes.

Saturated fat and the demonisation of cholesterol

At the time when the US township of Roseto was under investigation because life seemed almost too healthy for its citizens, a major epidemic of heart disease was spreading across America. In the nineteenth century, heart disease had been rare. But by the 1950s it was the number one reason for Americans to die, and although numbers are reducing, it still is today.

Researchers began associating saturated fat in the diet with increased levels of cholesterol in the bloodstream early in the twentieth century, at first by feeding animal fat to laboratory rabbits. They further established a correlation between having high cholesterol and an increased risk of heart disease. Thus, the following causal relationship was established: saturated fat, they surmised, raises cholesterol. This in turn causes heart disease. So, as a result, saturated fat must be largely responsible for heart disease.

Although no laboratory research on humans supported this (and rabbits, being vegetarians, are hardly a good indicator), repetition of the correlation gradually got this mantra established as fact. In this connection, we should heed the words of Daniel Kahnemann, the Nobel-prize-winning author of *Thinking Fast and Thinking Slow*:[182] 'A reliable way to make people believe in falsehoods is frequent repetition, because familiarity is not easily distinguished from truth. Authoritarian institutions and marketers have always known this fact'.

In 1977, this so-called 'diet-heart hypothesis' became US public policy and was officially endorsed by the Dietary Guidelines Advisory Committee – even though it had not been proven to be true. Doing something based on this hypothesis was considered to be in the public interest. Yet even today, when it has been shown that these initial assumptions were wrong, most people (including many doctors,

---

182 Kahnemann, 2011, p.62.

nutritionists and most of the diet industry) still hold on to this untruth as a well-established fact. That's why you most likely believe that you should avoid saturated fat in order to reduce heart disease risk. When I began my investigations, it was my belief too. But now I am convinced that it is not only untrue but that some of us are getting ill by eating too little fat; particularly too little saturated fat. As we have seen, the so-called healthy oils that we eat a lot of – both at home and especially in processed meals – are also gradually becoming accepted as being detrimental to our health. The Icelandic researcher, Kris Gunnars, has a well-put-together site[183] which aims to reveal all there is to know about fact-based nutrition. His article on the toxic nature of vegetable oils[184] is particularly informative.

The outstanding fact remains that there is no serious experimental evidence linking saturated fat to heart disease. And the assumption that eating food containing cholesterol will raise your blood cholesterol levels is plainly untrue, even if it had been important in the first place. Much of the nutrition research that I dug up was based on questionable correlation (and correlation does not equal causation) or demonstrated poor statistical levels of significance. However, the **Framingham Heart Study**[185] stands out as a well-run study. Based in a small community situated not far from Boston, Massachusetts, the Framingham Study followed (and continues to follow) fifteen thousand people over three generations and has provided much good solid and reliable information. Even in the 1990s, their findings demonstrated that cholesterol in the diet had no correlation with heart disease – but at the time, they were ignored.

The infamous 'diet-heart hypothesis', stating that eating foods rich in cholesterol leads to heart disease, was even criticised by Ancel Keys later on in his life. He is, by the way, the man considered by most to be the originator of this hypothesis. In 1997, he went on record as saying:[186] 'There's no connection whatsoever between the cholesterol in food and

183 See www.authoritynutrition.com
184 Gunnars, 2013.
185 Framingham Heart Study, n.d. (2).
186 See Feldman and Marks, 2006, Chapter 4: *The Great Cholesterol Myth*.

cholesterol in the blood. And we've known that all along. Cholesterol in the diet doesn't matter at all unless you happen to be a chicken or a rabbit'.

Keys was referring back to that research work on chickens and rabbits from 1920, which did establish such a relationship. But, as noted, because rabbits and chickens are mostly vegetarian, they hardly provide the right test-beds for establishing such a linkage. An increasing number of researchers now believe the primary cause of heart disease is inflammation and the related oxidative stress, but cholesterol still bears the brunt of the official blame. Let's return to the Framingham Heart Study and note the words of its director, William Castelli:[187] 'cholesterol levels by themselves reveal little about a patient's coronary artery disease risk'. In fact, he goes further: 'In Framingham, Mass., the more saturated fat one ate, the more cholesterol one ate, the *more calories one ate,* the lower the person's serum cholesterol' (Dr Castelli's italics).

He couldn't state it more plainly, could he? And yet supermarket aisles and processed food packaging still tout 'reduced cholesterol' as a benefit, often linking it with lower heart disease or even weight loss. Frederick Stare, the founder of the nutrition department at Harvard University and former American Heart Association member, was an early proponent of the lipid hypothesis (meaning that dietary fat leads to heart disease). In 1973, he was advocating:[188] 'a reduction in saturated fat and cholesterol content of dairy products; a reduction of saturated fat, cholesterol and calorie content of baked goods and a reduction of the use of egg yolk in foods'. Yet later on in his life he decreed that a little cholesterol was no bad thing and that the American Medical Association was unnecessarily scaring the public. He stated:[189] 'The cholesterol factor is of minor importance as a risk factor in CVD (cardiovascular disease). Of far more importance are smoking, hypertension, obesity, diabetes, insufficient physical activity, and stress'.

It's important to remember just how important cholesterol is for our bodies and, in particular, our brains. Your brain, more than half of which

187 Castelli, 1992.
188 Stare, 1973.
189 Stare et al., 1989.

consists of fat, may weigh in at around 3% of your total body weight, yet it contains round 25% of the total cholesterol found in your body. There is even research linking higher levels of cholesterol with improved memory function in older people.

Two further studies are worth quoting from in this context. First, the **Honolulu Heart Program**,[190] which followed eight thousand participants and published a report in 2001:[191] 'Long-term persistence of low cholesterol concentration actually increases the risk of death. Thus, the earlier the patients start to have lower cholesterol concentrations, the greater the risk of death'. Second, the huge **Japanese Lipid Intervention Trial**, with over forty-seven thousand participants:[192] 'The highest death rate observed was among those with lowest cholesterol (under 160mg/dl); lowest death rate observed was with those whose cholesterol was between 200-259mg/dl'.

Put in simple English: those with the lowest cholesterol had the highest death rate, and those with cholesterol levels that would today be called 'dangerous' had the lowest death rate.

As you can see, not only do high total levels of cholesterol not cause heart disease, but low cholesterol can actually be dangerous to your health. So this is beginning to add support to the idea that we toss out the vegetable oil and start eating butter and eggs again! But more on that as we continue. Let's start by developing and using new and positive language for cholesterol.

So … cholesterol is good for me?

To start with, because most human cholesterol (about 85%) is produced by your liver, you can effectively switch the production of cholesterol on and off – depending on whether it is supplemented by enough in the foods you eat. This means that whether you eat cholesterol-rich food or not is rather irrelevant. The medical textbooks tell us that

---

190 National Heart, Lung, and Blood Institute, 2005.
191 Schatz et al., 2001.
192 Mabuchi et al., 2002.

there are a number of important roles that cholesterol plays in your body, including:

- compensating for changes in membrane fluidity;

- promoting the production of the sex hormones testosterone, oestrogen, and progesterone;

- providing a building block for vitamin D and steroid hormones;

- acting as an antioxidant;

- aiding digestion by helping your liver make bile acids; and

- protecting your skin, making it suppler (did you know that cholesterol is added as an ingredient in many moisturizers to protect your skin from damage?).

Yet most of us are still conditioned to think that cholesterol will lead to the clogging of arteries and that we need to reduce levels by any means possible to avoid developing cardiovascular disease. Repeated messaging and clever advertising have combined to create a false picture of fats piling up in our arteries – much as fat can clog the waste pipe under a sink. The reality is quite different. It is the calcification and resultant thickening of your artery walls that are the real problem worth tackling. This hardening of the arteries is considered to be an inevitability of old age but is linked to the usual suspects of diabetes, obesity, environmental factors and poor diet (together with all its many interpretations).

Most of us have now learned that the so-called HDL is the good cholesterol while LDL is the bad type. It's an over-simplification, but it has its roots firmly anchored in reality. Interestingly, there is one food which has been shown to increase your levels of healthy HDL. That, ironically to some, is saturated fat. There is no drug on the market which can achieve such results, although admittedly, stopping smoking also generally sees a positive impact on HDL levels. Eating more saturated fat has also been shown to increase the size of your LDL particles (which is also considered to be a good thing, though difficult to measure in regular blood tests). Most nutrition experts, however, have ignored all this research because it doesn't quite fit with the other eating guidelines they prescribe. There'd be too much back-tracking necessary.

Taking a pharmaceutical approach and bearing in mind that so many people experience lower cholesterol levels by taking statins these days, Dr Darrel Francis of Imperial College London made the following comment in an interview published by *Medscape* in July 2014:[193] 'The HDL-raising concept does not seem to be beneficial in any of the statin-era trials, but it doesn't mean that any therapy that raises HDL will never work. For all we know, the LDL reduction might be doing the trick. So I am a bit pessimistic about the focus on HDL. I think if we're going to look at things, we might as well look at LDL cholesterol. That's where we've seen the most success'.

Hardly a ringing endorsement for statins! And when it comes to women, most are unaware that a low-fat diet may increase their risk for heart disease. In comments published back in 2004, Robert Knopp and Barbara Retzlaff still spoke of a 'saturated fat paradox'.[194] But perhaps it's time that we accepted that it is not a paradox but indeed a clear statement of fact. The exaggerated decreases in HDL cholesterol concentrations that he and his colleagues noted with the consumption of a low-fat diet, particularly in women, were highly significant. Commenting on the different effects of diet on lipoprotein physiology and cardiovascular disease risk, Knopp and Retzlaff said in their article's conclusion:[195] 'These effects include the paradox that a high-fat, high-saturated fat diet is associated with diminished coronary artery disease progression in women with the metabolic syndrome, a condition that is epidemic in the United States'.

In spite of all the research, supermarkets promote shopping aisles loaded with cholesterol-lowering spreads. In the UK, the NHS continues

---

193 O'Riordan, 2014. The interview related to research by Dr Francis and colleagues – see Keene et al., 2014.

194 Knopp and Retzlaff, 2004.

195 Idem.

to say on its website that:[196] 'High cholesterol ... increases your risk of serious health conditions'. Those readers still in doubt should take a look at Dr Donald Miller's 2015 article in *The Journal of American Physicians and Surgeons.*[197] His summary is outspoken, but as Emeritus Professor of Surgery and former Chief of Cardiothoracic Surgery at the University of Washington's School of Medicine, it deserves respect: 'It is becoming increasingly clear that the cholesterol/heart hypothesis is a fallacy of modern medicine. In the future, medical historians may liken the prescribing of statins to lower blood cholesterol with the old medical practice of bloodletting. Taking that vital substance out of the body is comparable to today's practice of blocking production of cholesterol, an equally vital component, with drugs'.

Although our prime subject matter here is cholesterol, it would be wrong to leave the subject without a comment on the oft-held suspicion that higher fat (particularly saturated fats) might promote cancer. In this context, it might be surprising to learn that as far back as 1987, the epidemiologist Walter Willett of the Harvard School of Public Health (who now chairs the Department of Nutrition) had found fat consumption not to be positively linked to breast cancer among the nearly ninety thousand nurses whom he had been following for five years in the Nurses' Health Study.[198] What he found was precisely the opposite; the greater the proportion of fat the nurses ate (and in particular saturated fat), the less likely they were to get breast cancer. After fourteen years of study, Willett reported that his team had found 'no evidence' that a reduction in fat overall – nor of any particular kind of fat – decreased the risk of breast cancer. Saturated fat actually appeared protective, and the results held true even as the women aged. As you well know by now, epidemiology studies (aka correlation) cannot demonstrate causation, but they can be used to show the absence of a correlation. Hence, it's pretty safe to assume that dietary fat in your diet does not lead to cancer. On balance, maybe you now agree that it most probably has a protective effect in general.

196 NHS, 2015 (2).
197 Miller, 2015.
198 Willett et al., 1987. See also Colditz, 1991.

Modern wheat and allergies – what's gone wrong?

Dieticians and government guidelines continue to say that whole wheat is an essential part of a 'balanced' diet, yet others say that wheat of any kind promotes heavier bodies and disease. What's going on?

As you may well have read, the flourishing paleo movement, which draws inspiration from earlier hunter-gatherer societies, shies away from all cereal crops. But humans have been consuming wheat, to varying extents, since arable farming began over ten thousand years ago. Modern genetics is suggesting that we adapt to new foodstuffs rather faster than the Darwinian school initially led us to believe. After all, even the Bible refers positively to the eating of your daily bread, and that's getting on for two thousand years old. Somehow, it just doesn't seem to make sense to blame wheat for so many of our new diet-related diseases. Yet it seems that some of us have adapted better than others.

Geneticists now inform us that it is a similar story when it comes to digesting milk, which has also only been drunk in larger quantities during the last few thousand years. Some of us possess all the necessary genes to cope with lactose, while some do not – not yet, that is. Others without the necessary genetic adaptation have what is called 'lactose sensitivity'.

Plants, like any other living thing, need to survive. Being immobile and stuck in the ground, they had to develop defence mechanisms against being eaten by insects and other animals. Their DIY pesticide strategy was designed to protect them by causing intestinal distress to their predators. That is why most older cultures (and medieval recipes) call for the soaking of grains prior to their consumption – simply because this starts the sprouting process and makes them more digestible. In the modern times in which we live, humans don't do this.

The funny thing is that the highest density of the anti-nutrient toxins can be found in the outer layers of the grain, but we are advised to eat whole-grain breads to help our digestion because of the fibre – as you can imagine, we should probably be doing just the opposite.

Gluten, phytates and lectins are the major toxic culprits, with gluten being famously the one that so many people want to avoid these days. Coming from the Latin word for glue, gluten is a protein found in grains like wheat, barley and rye. When you eat it, gluten enters the small intestine undigested, where it can cause irritation – mainly because it creates inflammation. This is associated with all sorts of health conditions including IBS, thyroid issues, neurological problems and pain disorders.

Then we get to phytates, which are powerful chelators. This means that they bind together with minerals, helping remove them from your body. People sometimes write that the phytates in grains remove other minerals from your body too, but in fact they only remove what is in the grain itself. In doing so, they (ironically) remove many of the much-hyped good vitamins and minerals found in wholemeal breads and oatmeal (which contains phytates but no gluten – unless it's been processed with other cereals).

Lectins, found in all plants and animal products, are sticky in nature and help bind together carbohydrates – but this means that they can sometimes attach themselves to the intestinal lining. Also known as anti-nutrients, they are often a greater culprit than gluten in causing upset stomachs and bloating. Even after fermentation or a good preparatory soaking before cooking, they can be resistant to breakdown. What's worse is that they bio-accumulate in your body, causing a cornucopia of health issues – from promoting leptin resistance (which, as we know, contributes to obesity) through to being toxic to your immune system.

When it comes down to it, let's remember that grains are simply seeds that don't want to be digested. If you eat them, they want to be excreted whole – that's how, in nature, they get spread around by birds and other animals. Our ancestors seemed to know this instinctively, and grain always went through an extensive pre-preparation phase. You can still observe this in more 'primitive' societies today; in Central Africa, millet is still soaked to the point of fermentation before being cooked.

So ... should we avoid wheat and other gluten-containing cereals totally? Although some of us are well-adapted and some less so, on balance, we should all reduce the amount of these seeded carbs that we eat. They certainly haven't helped us grow taller. Interestingly, they've not helped our brains either!

Smaller brains?

According to John Hawks of the University of Wisconsin,[199] over the past twenty thousand years, the average volume of the human male brain has decreased from 1,500 cubic centimetres to 1,350 (the female brain has shrunk by about the same proportion). 'I'd call that major downsizing in an evolutionary eyeblink,' he says.

Although theories as to why the human brain is shrinking are all over the place, it is clear that the *Homo Sapiens* with the biggest brains lived twenty to thirty thousand years ago in Central and Southern Europe. Called the Cro-Magnons, they had barrel chests, and large, jutting jaws with enormous teeth – so their larger brains have often been attributed to physical rather than mental strength.

Some scientists think that modern humans are simply getting dumber; others say that our internal wiring has become more efficient and that we are now quicker and more agile thinkers because of that. Some directly link smaller brains to the rise of farming and the increased use of cereal crops (when feeding ourselves and our animals). Still others believe that we have 'tamed' ourselves in the same way that we domesticated sheep, pigs, and cattle – all of which have smaller brains than their wild forebears. Domesticated breeds demonstrate a 10-15% reduction in brain size but also possess a more graceful stature with smaller teeth, flatter faces and a more striking range of colouration and hair type. Compared to many wild animals, domesticated ones also grow

199 Hawks, 2013.

floppier ears and curly tails. Apart from those two traits, the features shared by domesticated animals make them sound a lot like us!

But putting that aside and getting back to the subject matter, although we cannot precisely say why brains are smaller today, the old 'correlation is not causation' factor can show us one thing: namely that the consumption of so many cereal products has not helped our brains maintain their size – let alone assisted them in getting bigger!

Allergies and food intolerances

Today's levels of allergies and food intolerances have reached new heights; almost everyone knows someone with an allergy or food-related problem. Yet Great-Grandma's generation hardly knew of such things. And it's here that we must acknowledge that the wheat we now cook with is quite different from the way it was just fifty years ago.

First; we process it quite differently. Automated techniques of grain processing first developed in the late nineteenth century now make it possible to create massive amounts of refined wheat at a low cost. This white flour, combined with the ready availability of sugar, has fuelled many aspects of baking - even what we call 'haute-cuisine' today, with so many sauces, cakes and pastries being based on the French way of creating them. After all, even a light cheese soufflé is based on a roux sauce, which has been thickened with processed and refined white flour.

It was the ability to industrially separate the bran and germ (containing many nutritious, and yet also toxic, components of the grain) away from the endosperm that left us with easy accessibility to these starchy carbs we now enjoy in the form of white flour. This process led to a reduction in nutrient density, but it also created white flour's ability to spike blood sugar very fast.

Shortcutting the soaking, sprouting and fermenting processes to make pre-packaged, pre-sliced Wonder Bread was augmented by the elimination of slow-rise yeast in the baking process. Yet it was just these healthy but time-consuming procedures that contributed to the reduction in the amount of anti-nutrients (such as phytic acid and lectins) in bread, while making the other nutrients more accessible.

Today's flour is also often bleached with chlorine before being baked using a cocktail of quick-rise yeast and raising chemicals – in conjunction with the Chorleywood bread-making process – to create rolls and breads of all shapes and forms. Small amounts of real yeast (or yeast flavour) are now sometimes added to improve the taste – after the event, so to speak! So, if we were summarising, it is clear that the bread, cookies and cakes we enjoy today are very different from the traditionally prepared breads and pastries that have been a staple part of our diet for thousands of years.

But this evolution is not just about the manufacturing and processing of flour, breads and pastries. Going back in time, we used to sow ancient, simpler varieties of wheat containing fewer chromosomes – such as emmer, einkorn, khorasan (known as kamut) and, more recently, spelt. Today, what is sown is mostly a high-yield semi-dwarf variety. This was developed by cross-breeding and simple but efficient genetic manipulation in the 1960s. With shorter stems, it is also less likely to be blown over in strong winds, making it more economical in other ways – but its nutrient and protein composition has changed more than we ever considered.

Organic wheat? Do 'older' grains make better bread?

The world has produced a lot more grain since the so-called Green Revolution of the 1960s. As a result, it is argued that many people have been freed from famine. But quantity does not always equal quality. Let's take a look at some data from the Broadbalk experiment, famous because it is the longest-running agricultural experiment in the world. Analyses of crop samples from their base at Rothamsted Research Station, situated near London, show that the levels of essential micro-nutrients in wheat grain, which remained consistent from their start-up in 1844 to the late 1960s, have since then continued to decline.[200]

In the 1960s and '70s, traditional long-straw wheat varieties were phased out in favour of higher-yielding semi-dwarf varieties. But

---

200 Fan et al., 2008.

compared to the old long-straw varieties, modern dwarf wheat grain carries on average 20-30% less zinc, iron, copper and magnesium. For zinc, a critical human nutrient, the decline has accelerated during the most recent five years, providing further evidence that organic farmers need to also concentrate on the seed grain they use, rather than just the healthy and sustainable growing conditions.

Coeliac disease

Coeliac disease is the most severe form of gluten intolerance; the immune system in the gut mistakenly assumes that gluten proteins are foreign invaders and so it mounts an attack. Unfortunately, the immune system doesn't just attack the gluten proteins – it attacks the gut lining itself. This is what leads to leaky gut, inflammation and numerous other harmful effects. Sufferers must avoid all (and can be sensitive to the tiniest) trace elements.

For reasons which are debated, the incidence of coeliac disease has increased about four-fold during the past forty-five years, now affecting about 1% of people in Western societies. We must not confuse this with gluten sensitivity, which is different and more common, affecting a much larger group (estimated at 6-8% of people around the world).

Gluten is actually not a single protein but a family of different proteins, and only some of them are recognized by the immune system of coeliac patients. One of those proteins is called Glia-α9, and it seems to be particularly problematic. The level of this protein is significantly higher in modern wheat, and this could the main reason why modern wheat is worse for coeliac patients than older varieties of wheat.

There are, as mentioned, alternatives to modern wheat. In several (admittedly small) group studies, einkorn has been shown to have few harmful effects – the gluten from einkorn causes significantly less adverse reactions than modern gluten. Einkorn is a historic variety of wheat; it has been grown for over five thousand years and contains just two sets of chromosomes. Other earlier forms of wheat such as emmer, kamut and durum wheat are also descendants of early wild grasses, usually having four sets of chromosomes. Modern hybrid wheat has six. Using earlier wheat varieties is not the only factor in aiding digestion. Traditionally made sourdough bread has also been shown to cause less of a reaction in coeliac patients than today's industrialised bread does.

To be clear, I am not for a moment suggesting that coeliac sufferers should immediately try out traditional bread-making methods. But the increased auto-immune reaction in the gut caused by modern wheat and manufacturing methods may well be why coeliac disease and gluten sensitivity are on the rise. Modern wheat certainly contains an increased proportion of problematic glutens, and enough studies show that older wheat varieties don't cause a reaction in coeliac patients. It's an area where further research is urgently needed.

Stick with Einkorn and Kamut

There are many skeptics out there who simply refuse to believe that something as basic as wheat might be problematic or even harmful to 'normal' non-coeliacs too. Yet a growing number of people suffer from IBS – and they blame everything from the effects of ibuprofen to heightened stress levels when maybe, just maybe, modern wheat is playing a role. The following research work carried out by the University of Florence in 2014 shows pretty clearly the benefits of using traditional kamut flour, at least on Italians:[201]

The researchers set out to examine the effect of a replacement diet using organic, semi-whole-grain (ancient) wheat on irritable bowel syndrome (IBS) symptoms and related inflammatory/biochemical parameters.

A double-blind randomised cross-over trial was performed using twenty participants (13 females and 7 males, aged 18–59 years), each classified as having IBS (Irritable Bowel Syndrome)-related problems. The participants received bread, pasta, biscuits and crackers made either from ancient wheat (khorasan, known as kamut) or modern dwarf wheat for a period of six weeks in a random order. Their IBS symptoms such as bloating, stomach pain and the ominous sounding 'problematic stool

---

201 Sofi et al., 2014.

consistency' were evaluated using two questionnaires and completed on a weekly basis. Blood analyses were also carried out at the beginning and end of each respective intervention period.

The results were clear-cut. When eating the ancient wheat products, patients experienced a significant decrease in the severity of their IBS symptoms, such as abdominal pain, bloating, dissatisfaction with stool consistency and tiredness. No significant difference was observed when feeding on modern wheat products. Similarly, patients reported a significant improvement in the severity of gastrointestinal symptoms after the ancient wheat intervention period, in terms of both the intensity and frequency of pain and their perceived quality of life. Their blood tests also showed a significant reduction in the circulating levels of pro-inflammatory cytokines and vascular endothelial growth factor after the use of ancient wheat products.

Although this sample was small, the results were overwhelmingly positive and point to significant improvements in both IBS symptoms and the inflammatory profile after the ingestion of ancient wheat products. The researchers are now embarking on a larger study.

Let's summarise: on a low-carb diet, you'll be wanting to skip the wheat flour entirely. But if the occasional slice of bread comes in handy (and I must admit to having some that I made, now pre-sliced in my freezer, which I very occasionally use for toast), buy or make a naturally fermented or sprouted bread made from one of the earlier and less sophisticated wheat types. I only bake using einkorn flour (recipe on the www.fatisourfriend.com website), but on my recent visit to Italy, I ate some bread made from local durum wheat, which they usually use for their pasta. Being someone who has experienced digestive problems when eating regular bread, I'm pleased to say that the experience was tasty and pleasing in all ways – but I only ate a little, and for me that required a lot of self-discipline!

Even though wheat (and the way we used to prepare it) may have been healthier in the past, today's wheat is different. So my advice is to avoid eating it; skip the sandwiches and the burger buns – and not just because they are high in insulin-provoking carbohydrates.

PART 7

SUMMARY

Remind me! Why ditch the sugars and starches? Why dial up the healthy fat?

Chances are that your friends are still pointing suspicious fingers at fat and desperately counting calories, so you may want to build up some convincing arguments for those coffee bar chats; they might think you're a bit crazy when you decide to eat 'high-fat, low-carb' like Katy did. This simple list reiterates why carbohydrates, rather than fats, are the problem.

If, on the other hand, you decide to give Katy's diet a try for a few weeks, I'm pretty confident that you will quickly develop all the proof that any of your friends might need – that being your own success story.

1. **Sugar and carbs raise your insulin levels.** Insulin is the hormone which causes you to store excess food as fat and also down-regulates how active you are. In excess, it interferes with hunger signalling from the leptin hormone to your brain and turns off your ability to burn fat. Sugar and carbs drive up insulin levels, whereas fat has little direct effect on insulin. That does not, sadly, mean that you can combine it with sugar (100% carbohydrate) and think you're better off!

2. **Low-carb, high-fat diets work** ... and have been shown to be effective in cases of 'diabesity' (insulin resistance). When tested against each other for twelve months, the low-carb, high-fat (LCHF) diet won out over two low-fat diet plans, namely Zone and Ornish.[202] Although low-fat diets did work for the minority of people who were insulin-sensitive, people in general found it easier to stick to the tastier low-carb, high-fat diet.

3. **Eating too much sugar is associated with disease.** When you measure consistently high sugar levels in people's blood, the

---

202 See Gardner et al., 2007.

higher blood sugar reading also correlates with an increased incidence of cancer, cardiovascular disease, and type-2 diabetes.

4. **Sugar and refined carbs are addictive; fat is not.** When you eat and digest sugar, for your body, it's almost as if you were taking cocaine or other addictive substances in terms of the brain pathways followed. What happens then is not down to a lack of self-control. Many overweight (and most obese) people are insulin-resistant; this blocks signalling by the leptin hormone, meaning their appetite control is disrupted. Dopamine levels will also go down, and since dopamine produced by your brain is part of the circuitry that makes you feel good and gives you self-confidence, this also affects your general sense of wellbeing. All this adds up to further stimulation of your 'need' for sugars and starches, which you go on to eat and drink in the form of highly processed carbs.

5. **Eating more saturated fats like butter, lard and coconut oil will improve your blood test results; sugar and carbs do the opposite.** The main reason that the nutrition establishment still gets upset about eating saturated fat is that it tends to raise LDL cholesterol, which used to be thought of as a sign of future heart disease. Now, we are better informed. Since saturated fat improves other blood markers such as triglycerides and HDL cholesterol, the earlier over-simplification is largely discredited. *If we had a drug that did what saturated fat achieves, many doctors would prescribe it.* Additionally, closer examination of related LDL readings has shown no increase in Apolipoprotein B, the so-called smaller dense lipoproteins which are more strongly associated with poor health. If anything, they help increase the size of LDL cholesterol, making the higher reading a positive.[203]

6. **Saturated fats don't easily get damaged by higher cooking temperatures.** Humans have been safely eating saturated fats for

203 See Sigurdsson, 2015.

hundreds of thousands of years. Whereas modern, industrially produced unsaturated fats like corn, soy and sunflower oil give off toxic side-effects (which you breathe in and eat) and go rancid more quickly; butter, coconut oil and lard do not.

7. **Saturated fats from dairy and meat contain lots of naturally occurring fat-soluble vitamins and minerals.** Eating such fats also helps you digest these vitamins and minerals, forming a more resilient body and allowing calcium to be effectively incorporated into bone. Incidentally, dairy from grass-fed cows is measurably more nutritious than that from 'conventionally' raised animals (the same goes for eggs from outside-reared chickens), being especially rich in mineral nutrients such as zinc, iron and phosphorous, and in fat-soluble vitamins such as vitamins A, E and K2.[204]

Let's summarise: If you regularly eat high-fat foods that also contain a high level of processed carbs, as we so often do in our Western diet, then things are not going to go well for you. Big Mac meals, blueberry muffins and Snickers bars will never contribute to a healthy diet. But if you cook and prepare foods using fresh ingredients, fat in most of its forms is just fine. You do need to avoid the industrially produced seed oils like corn, soy and sunflower, but saturated fats such as butter, lard and coconut oil do you good, as does olive oil.

In absolute terms, we all have somewhat different tolerances for carbs and that's why there is no 'one-size-fits-all' solution. The younger you are, then usually the more insulin-sensitive you are, so you can safely eat higher levels of carbs; but with too much, you too start slowing down, burning fat less efficiently and putting on weight. Statistically speaking, if you are an older female, both overweight and stressed out through work and/or family, then you are high up on the 'insulin-resistant' list. You almost certainly need to eat fewer foods containing carbohydrates in your diet – especially sugar. It may seem unfair that just when you feel

204 See Daley et al., 2010.

that you've earned that chocolate bar in the evening, you are told you cannot have it (unless it's 85% pure chocolate, of course). You could, of course, try traditional calorie restriction to lose weight. But what you'll end up doing is simply masking the problem. Any protein you eat beyond your daily requirements will pass through you or be turned into glucose anyway (gluconeogenesis), which defeats the purpose. But increasing your fat intake will help you lose weight and improve your blood markers because you will feel fuller and less hungry.

A reminder of foods you should avoid – especially sugar

There is a growing body of opinion which supports cutting out ready-made, commercial foods and switching to home cooking. That being said, we need to get more specific to provide everyday guidance. So, in no particular order, the main 'diabesity' culprits are:

- Almost everything behind the counter at Starbucks, Costa etc.!

- Sugar, particularly fructose (especially high-fructose corn syrup). This includes fruit juices.

- Cereal grains, especially wheat flour.

- Omega-6-rich industrial seed oils such as corn, sunflower, safflower, soybean, etc. (including most deep fried food from take-aways, and potato chips).

When it comes to sweetness, you'll remember that normal white sugar contains a 50:50 mix of glucose and fructose and that glucose, in smaller doses, is an important nutrient. Fructose, however, is another story. Although fructose is found naturally in fruits and vegetables, it is infamously also the major constituent in cheap, industrially produced high-fructose corn syrup (HFCS), so the quantities we eat are increasing. Glucose, which is still marketed in pure tablet form to help diabetics who are experiencing hypoglycaemia (low blood glucose), is rapidly absorbed into the bloodstream. Fructose, however, goes straight to the liver, where it is converted to fat. In excess, it can lead to non-alcoholic fatty liver disease (NAFLD), which undermines your body's energy reserves and is directly linked to both diabetes and obesity. More people today suffer from NAFLD than suffer from the more well-known alcohol-related condition. Dr Robert H. Lustig, who wrote the *New York Times* bestseller,

Fat Chance, explains that fructose is toxic and that it:[205] 'causes damage, provides no benefit and is sent directly to the liver to be detoxified (and turned into fat) so that it doesn't harm the body'.

Fructose can also form up to ten times as much of the toxic compounds known as Advanced Glycation End-Products (AGEs) than glucose does. These damage DNA, speed up the ageing process, cause high blood pressure and lead to kidney disease. It is OK to eat fruit in moderation, even though it's sweet(!), but you are advised to stop drinking fructose-rich fruit juices – which means definitely dropping the morning OJ. Also stop the sweet sodas, and – above all – avoid foods wherever you can which include HFCS on the label! For the record, a large-scale study of nurses recently published by the British Medical Association,[206] which involved researchers from the UK, USA and Singapore, found that people who ate whole fruit (especially blueberries, grapes and apples) were less likely to get type-2 diabetes than those who drank fruit juice.

Wheat, corn, rice, barley and oats have become the staple crops of our modern Western diet. Known collectively as cereal crops, they are at the heart of the low-fat, high-carbohydrate diet agenda promoted by government bodies responsible for dietary guidelines – and, interestingly, still favoured by most diabetes associations around the world. As an observation, their edicts and recommendations inevitably play on the perception that while white flour may not be particularly nutritious, whole grains are healthy. A large (but difficult to quantify) number of us struggle with digesting these grains, but what you might not know is that many animals, including monkeys and apes, have never adapted to eating cereal grains (grasses, in their original form) either. We humans have only been eating them for the past ten thousand years or so, and even when they are refined and processed, the natural defences developed by these plants and grasses include the production of toxins which can damage the human stomach lining, making digestion more difficult and hindering the absorption of proteins.

---

205 Lustig, 2013.
206 Muraki et al., 2013.

A reminder of foods you should eat – and where to find low-carb recipes

If you have decided to give up bread, cakes and sugary snacks, you have taken a big step forward towards rediscovering a healthier you. But there is still a danger that you focus too much on what you can't eat and what you can no longer do (such as go to fast-food restaurants) rather than bringing into view the vast cornucopia of food and drink that is available to you. As natural worriers, we too often see the world from a 'glass half-empty' perspective. Thankfully, though, the World Wide Web has come to our rescue, and makes this so much easier for us than it would have been just a few years ago.

I encourage you to start with a look through some of my recipes at www.fatisourfriend.com – but there are also many, many low-carb cooking sites on the web these days, full of appetising creations. Remember that low-carb is not no-carb, and you will need to find the balance that works for you – some people continue the diet and eat a few small salad potatoes on the side, and some choose not to. You can also safely visit any of the so-called paleo diet websites and read from the vast number of recipes they also have on offer. A word of warning: most paleo dieters use no dairy – so, in fact, you have much more choice than they do. Their mantra, as genetic expert Tim Spector reflects, is: 'Our ancestors didn't eat like this, so we shouldn't'. This is because eating grains, milk, butter, yoghurt, cheese, coffee or alcohol only came into existence with farming, around ten thousand years ago. They argue that we have not, in a Darwinian sense, been able to adapt to these foodstuffs. However, recent evidence published in the magazine *Nature*[207] suggests that major changes to our genes can occur in just a few hundred generations. They showed that although light skin pigmentation in Europeans was already common in the Bronze Age (that's four to five thousand years ago), lactose tolerance – the ability to digest milk easily – was rare. Around

---

207 Allentoft et al., 2015.

75% of modern Europeans now have this gene, which allows them to drink milk without feeling sick – but only 5% possessed this ability then.

We can adapt faster than paleo dieters would have you believe, particularly because sometimes it's our bacterial genes that need to change. Those in our guts need to try and respond rapidly to changes in our diet; given that they produce a new generation every thirty minutes, they are pretty good at doing just that.

I, too, believe that we can learn from our forebears, but I have come to believe that the paleo approach is too anchored in the past. That's not to say that some of their recipes don't taste fantastic – and, by definition, they are invariably low-carb. When it comes down to it, we need to keep our gut microbes as healthy as we can, and dietary diversity is the key. The Weston A. Price Foundation[208] espouses a more pragmatic and relevant dietary approach which is similar in many ways to the dietary advice listed in this book. Weston Price was a dentist who originally travelled the world in the earlier part of the twentieth century looking for non-industrialised communities and comparing their teeth with the degeneration he was finding among his US patients. Noting the healthy jawbones and invariably straight teeth, free from decay, that he found on his travels, he became more and more convinced that the dental caries and deformation he was seeing back home were linked to nutritional deficiencies.

With the vast selection of meats, fish, dairy and vegetables you have to choose from, combined with the protective power of saturated fat and some small portions of fruit, you can trim your weight, gain energy and also reduce your blood sugar levels. Your conventionally trained doctor may not be an advocate of this approach at the start of this process – but if he or she is anything like mine or Katy's, they will appreciate the slimmer and healthier end result.

Let's leave our final words to some bankers; the analysts at Credit Suisse. I think it's fair to say that they have no vested interest one way or another in this matter. They examined the role that fat plays as an ingredient in foods of all kinds around the world, and checked their

208 www.westonaprice.org

facts against all available scientific material, wanting to provide a firm footing for their investor community when looking at future trends. Their conclusion, published in September 2015, was that:[209] 'Saturated fat has not been a driver of obesity: fat does not make you fat. At current levels of consumption, the most likely culprit behind growing obesity level of the world population is carbohydrates'.

On the subject of saturated fat itself, they stated: 'One of the biggest myths in nutrition is that saturated fat intake above a certain level – say 10% based on most dietary guidelines – significantly increases your risk of heart attack. This conclusion that has held for almost half a century is inconsistent with the wealth of epidemiological data or scientific evidence in the form of clinical randomized trials. Plenty of research funding has been earmarked to study and back this hypothesis, yet we cannot find a single research paper written in the last ten years that supports this conclusion. On the contrary, we can find at least 20 studies that dismiss this hypothesis'.

I rest my case. Fat, at least when you choose it in a wise and informed way, can be your very best friend.

---

209 Credit Suisse Research Institute, 2015.

PART 8

MY PERSONAL ROSETO INVESTIGATION

Introduction

In this final chapter, you will find the more detailed review of my search to discover whether the 'old-fashioned' diet eaten by Rosetans up until the 1960s was having a positive, protective effect on their health or whether it was social cohesion alone that led to their healthier hearts.

Students of Sociology learn that the 'Roseto Effect' is the phenomenon by which a close-knit community experiences a reduced rate of heart disease. No-one can prove either hypothesis one way or the other, but I certainly came to the conclusion that their fat-rich diet was helping them stay healthy for longer. Although much lower in carbohydrates than the standard American diet, which is around 55% or so carbs, there was no truly low-carb approach to their pattern of eating, even if it was relatively high in fat – but there again, the Rosetans were not trying to diet. They felt no need to go on diets, and I would like to think that just like their forebears in Puglia, Italy, the community of Roseto was primarily healthy because of the fresh and locally sourced food that they ate. If they had stuck to those principles and kept more of a sense of community, maybe they would still be living longer and healthier lives, just as their relatives in Southern Italy still do.

Why did the inhabitants of one small town in Pennsylvania live such long and healthy lives? Family values, nourishing food or perhaps both?

Roseto was unique in one very obvious way; it had been inaugurated as the very first 100% Italian borough in the United States of America – thanks to the official stamp of approval granted by Judge Henry Scott on January 2nd, 1912. Originally settled in the 1890s by immigrants, the community named it after the poor rural village of Roseto Valfortore, from where most of the settlers originated. That original Roseto Valfortore is still to be found in Puglia, South Eastern Italy, about 100 kilometres east of Naples. With recent government and European Union assistance (as I saw with my own eyes in September 2014), it has become more successful than the village those early settlers left over one hundred years ago.

But for now, let's go back to Pennsylvania at a time of growth and great hope for the future – the 1960s. Back then, Roseto already enjoyed a reputation as a friendly town, being both welcoming to guests and representing the best of old-fashioned family values. These were anchored in firm societal foundations – those being the Italian traditions of cultural values and community. What drew medical interest in Roseto, however, was its extraordinary death statistics. Rosetans lived longer, healthier lives than other Americans. Back then, Rosetans died of heart attacks less than half as often as other Americans. Yet when examining the daily lives of the Rosetans, the medical community considered that precisely the opposite should have been the case. Its residents should have been dying at a decidedly younger age than average Americans, they thought. Their mix of poor diet, too much wine, hard physical labour at the local slate mines and just the same high levels of smoking as elsewhere across the States hardly augured well for a longer, healthier life. The town was also visibly in the early stages of decline. It had faded somewhat since its heyday in the 1940s, when the main street, Garibaldi Avenue, had featured three butcher's shops, seven grocery stores, two bakers and eight bars or restaurants. Local industries weren't faring too well either. The slate mines and earlier weaving industries were slowly dying out, and – just to bring things up to date – you would easily see how things have continued to change if you were to pay a visit today. Suburban commuters, satellite dishes, fenced-in yards and expensive cars make Roseto look like many other suburban townships. You will still find a barber's shop, a bakery and a single restaurant in the main street, but with the disappearance of the local industries the township has become, over time, a purely residential community. And oh yes – today, the health statistics mirror the American average. Malcolm Gladwell (whose book, *Outliers: The Story of Success*, was discussed in Part 4) was right; Roseto really was an outlier for a certain period of time in the middle of the last century. But why?

Joe Stampone, a relative of one of the founding fathers of the Roseto community in Pennsylvania, explained why early researchers were so intrigued:[210] 'Virtually no resident under fifty-five died of a heart attack; for men over sixty-five, the death rate from heart attack was half that of the United States as a whole; and the death rate from all causes was 35% lower than it should have been. There was no suicide, no alcoholism, no drug addiction and little crime to speak of. No one was on welfare and no one even suffered from peptic ulcers. These people died of old age, many of them in their eighties and nineties. That's it!'.

It simply defied logic that men, many of whom smoked and had spent a large proportion of their lives working in back-breaking – even dangerous – jobs such as those in the nearby slate quarries, would get home to face an evening meal of traditional Italian food accompanied by bottles of their locally made wine and still be so healthy. Their daily food represented a dietician's worst nightmare!

In *The Mystery of the Rosetan People*, Dr Rock Positano, another descendant of one of those founding fathers, listed why the immigrants'

---

210 Stampone, 2011.

lifestyles and diets were not the reason for their surprisingly good levels of health:[211] 'They smoked old-style Italian stogie cigars. Both sexes drank wine with seeming abandon. Rosetan men worked in such toxic environments as the nearby slate quarries … inhaling gases, dusts and other niceties. Rosetans fried their sausages and meatballs in lard. They ate salami, hard and soft cheeses all brimming with cholesterol'.

Observers also noted that the Rosetans could not afford the 'healthy' olive oil which was already being touted as a key ingredient in the wholesome Mediterranean diet gradually coming into vogue. And, as for how they looked, the medical investigators studying the population did not categorise the body shapes of Rosetans as being particularly slim; the unusual factor that they all shared was simply unusually strong and healthy hearts.

The lead investigator, Dr Stewart Wolf (whose work was considered briefly in Part 4) automatically tagged the Rosetan diet as being bad and unhealthy. It was so self-evident to him that the standard American diet was better than what they were eating that he quickly discounted what they consumed each day and began to search elsewhere for answers to this paradox. To start with, he looked at their family gene pools for unusual health tendencies and checked on the lives of other immigrants originating from Roseto, Valfortore in Italy. But it turned out that when living elsewhere across the States, they were no healthier than the average American. So genetic advantages were also removed from the list of the more obvious suspects leading to their longer lives.

Dr Wolf then examined the way healthcare was administered and even took samples of the local water supply – but it turned out to be identical to that piped in to the neighbouring towns of Nazareth and Bangor, which also shared the same hospital. So there were another two topics that he could cross off his list.

When all the evidence was in, the results led those examining the situation to develop the now well-documented and accepted theory known simply as the 'Roseto effect' – the phenomenon by which a close-knit community experiences a reduced rate of heart disease. In the words

---

211 Positano, 2008.

again of Dr Wolf (and colleagues), when attributing their lower heart disease rate entirely to reduced stress levels:[212] 'The community was very cohesive. There was no keeping up with the Joneses. Houses were very close together, and everyone lived more or less alike. Elderly were revered and incorporated into community life. Housewives were respected, and fathers ran the families'.

As Joe Stampone put it:[213] 'It was Roseto itself. The Rosetans (as they call themselves) visited each other on a daily basis, stopping to chat or cooking for each other in the back yard. Extended family clans were the norm, with three generations commonly living under the same roof. They went to Mass and saw the calming and unifying effect of the church. There were twenty-two civic associations in a town of less than two thousand people'.

---

212 Egolf et al., 1992.
213 Stampone, 2011.

Less stress and a positive attitude keeps you healthier?

Now, I would be the first to admire this old-fashioned (yet strangely enticing) way of living, and wholeheartedly agree that lower levels of stress do contribute to a healthier and longer life. Put in a modern historical context, there is now considerable independent research from newer sources that also goes to support this theory.

A 2006 study carried out by researchers at Carnegie University[214] demonstrated that a positive attitude can really affect our health over the years. They took 193 healthy adult volunteers and set out to make them ill! They administered nasal drops containing a cold or flu virus whilst at the same time assessing them for their emotional style. The emotional tendencies that the volunteers showed towards happiness and liveliness were contrasted with others' traits such as anxiousness, hostility or depressive tendencies.

As the volunteers developed their symptoms, mucus production was compared across the group, with significant and surprising results. The most emotionally positive of the volunteers produced less mucus, indicating that their emotional tendencies resulted in a demonstrable biological impact. They also showed fewer overall symptoms; indeed, fewer of them got sick than those volunteers with a more negative emotional style.

So a positive attitude to life can clearly help, and so too does the absence of stress; something apparently experienced by the inhabitants of that Rosetan community back in the 1960s. Research published in the *British Medical Journal* in 2012[215] showed that the risk of heart attacks or strokes increases by 20% when a person suffers from even low-level stress. According to that study, mortality rates from causes such as these escalate as a result of psychological distress, including anxiety and depression.

---

214 Cohen, 2006.
215 Russ et al., 2012.

So, by now you may not be surprised to know that studies also show increased survival rates for those cancer and HIV patients who have a strong social support network. A Yale university study[216] went further and asked 660 elderly people directly whether they agreed that we become less useful as we age. Over the years, they discovered that those with the most positive attitude to ageing lived on average seven and a half years longer than those with the most negative attitudes.

The Roseto effect was a pre-cursor to these studies, and this more recent research lends solid support to the essential premise. Levels of stress, your support network and having a positive outlook on life all contribute to your health and wellbeing. Up until now, today's generally held supposition that all of the Rosetans' healthy heart-related benefits can be explained purely in these sociological 'quality-of-life' terms has never really been questioned. Until today, that is – but we'll get to that very soon.

To sum things up: positive, happier people seem to live longer, healthier lives because they experience less stress; or a more nuanced interpretation could be that their personalities are less sensitive to the levels of stress they see and feel around them. One man's stress can undoubtedly be another's positive stimulus in certain situations. You may well take on a specific challenge and see it as something positive and uplifting; another person might consider that same challenge an unsettling risk; yet another might be even frightened at the very thought of it. In March of this year, the thrill-seeking centenarian Georgina Harwood went shark-diving in South Africa just two days after she had been sky-diving to celebrate her hundredth birthday!

We have all met people who just get on with things however bad they appear to be and others who get flustered at small changes to their daily routines. Those with a negative attitude are probably the ones who get angry or frustrated more easily – they're more likely to suffer from road rage! And it seems all too logical that their hearts suffer as a result.

But should we really believe that every single inhabitant of Roseto over the years was so positive towards life and so stress-free that, together

---

216 Levy et al., 2002.

with their strong sense of community, they were effectively equipped with stronger hearts?

Was it just their family-oriented lifestyle and their great community spirit which separated Roseto from the rest of the United States? Or did the use of lard, the lack of 'modern' oils and the abundant fresh vegetables play a role? It is worth remembering that the research in question was carried out in the 1960s but that those healthy men and women who were surveyed had grown up during the earlier decades of the twentieth century.

In *The Power of Clan: The Influence of Human Relationships on Heart Disease*[217] (a later report on studies by Dr Wolf and the sociologist John Bruhn, which covered the period of time from 1935 to 1984), the findings were clear: it was mutual respect and cooperation which contributed to the health and welfare of the community and its inhabitants. Yet when tracing back the history of Roseto, they also found out something interesting about the insular nature of their particular community. It appears that at the time, these early Italian immigrants were shunned by the English and Welsh who dominated this little corner of Eastern Pennsylvania. As a result, the Rosetans turned inward and, as Wolf and Bruhn noted in *The Power of Clan*:[218] 'radiated a kind of joyous team spirit as they celebrated religious festivals and family landmarks'. They truly did rediscover their Italian way of life in a very insular way, and were highly self-sufficient with farming and growing Italian staples such as vegetables and grapes.

During the 1960s (and even as late as 2007, when Malcolm Gladwell wrote *Outliers: The Story of Success*[219]), it was considered too ridiculous to even consider questioning whether what they ate could have been playing a positive role too; particularly since a doctor whose speciality was the digestive system was the lead investigator. Of course it wasn't helping at all! Their diet was:[220] 'grotesquely unhealthy; it consisted namely of too much red meat, lard, cholesterol, eggs, aged cheeses and wine'. Dr Wolf,

217 Wolf and Bruhn, 1993.
218 Idem.
219 Gladwell, 2008.
220 Bruhn and Wolf, 1979.

that original investigator, had dismissed the dietary factor out of hand. But today, when examining this decision, there is an interesting clue to be found when going back to his original reports and comparing them to the supposedly good dietary practices found elsewhere in America.

First, the context. We must bear in mind that by the 1960s, most Americans were already eating what's now often referred to as the standard American diet; largely carbohydrate-based, featuring ever-increasing quantities of processed seed oils, less fresh vegetables, less fibre, more processed meat (of the hot dog and hamburger variety), more sugar and more sodas (Coca-Cola and the like). Home cooking was already in decline, fast-food restaurants were booming, and at this time the whole of the United States of America was experiencing escalating levels of heart-related disease – even among younger people, particularly men; yet Roseto was not.

That potential clue, to be found in Dr Wolf's initial report, is a statement that:[221] '... a whopping 41% of their calories came from fat'. Much of it was meat-based and generally described as saturated fat. It would, incidentally, have contained relatively high levels of omega-3 fatty acids, since their animals were still primarily of the free-range type. In addition, they preferred using lard to corn oil.

The funny thing was, I had seen that figure of 41% in some recent research, and it had nothing to do with what they ate in Roseto. One of the few robust pieces of dietary research was carried out in Spain just a few years ago. Researchers followed a total of 7,447 men and women over a five-year period to assess whether a so-called Mediterranean diet was good for their hearts and whether adding more fat would change the findings.[222] All participants had symptoms which put them in a higher-risk category. These included type-2 diabetes, high blood pressure and their smoking habits. A daily dose of nuts or additional olive oil was added to the diet of two groups of the participants, and they left the third group with just low-fat guidelines and counselling (but no specific controls). Let's not forget that this was all within the context of a Spanish,

---

221 Gladwell, 2008, p.8.
222 Estruch et al., 2013.

Mediterranean-style diet, which is naturally richer in oily fish and fresh vegetables than most Westernised diets. Yet what happened was that they had to stop the test before the end of the fifth year, simply because the fattier diets were so much more beneficial. There was a 30% reduction in 'cardiovascular events' among those on the fattier dietary regimes. Interestingly, such diets contain relatively small amounts of omega-6 fats because the related cooking habits do not include much in the way of seed oils from corn, sunflower, soy, etc. And the dietary fat percentage enjoyed by the healthiest group of participants? Yes, you guessed right – it was indeed 41%. A coincidence, of course – but it made me think.

So rather than contributing negatively to their health, as Dr Wolf surmised, could the particular diet that they were enjoying have been protecting them? Could it have been adding to the quality of their lives? Could their diet have been part of the explanation of why they experienced such low levels of heart attacks and almost non-existent levels of strokes? Was this 'healthy' fat, when combined with fresh ingredients and traditional Italian cooking methods, part of their recipe for longer, healthier lives?

Conventional wisdom

Now when I said earlier that Dr Wolf 'dismissed the diet factor out of hand', that does not mean that he did not consider it as being potentially significant. His medical speciality (rather ironically) was the field of digestion, so (not surprisingly) a comprehensive dietary analysis was a key initial part of his investigation. As Malcolm Gladwell wrote:[223] 'Wolf's first thought was that the Rosetans must have held on to some dietary practices from the old world that left them healthier than other Americans. But he quickly realized that wasn't true. The Rosetans were cooking with lard, instead of the much healthier olive oil they used back in Italy. Pizza in Italy was a thin crust with salt, oil, and perhaps some tomatoes, anchovies or onions. Pizza in Pennsylvania was bread dough plus sausage, pepperoni, salami, ham and sometimes eggs. Sweets like biscotti and taralli used to be reserved for Christmas and Easter; now they were eaten all year round. When Wolf had dieticians analyse the typical Rosetan's eating habits, he found that a whopping 41 percent of their calories came from fat'.

Conventional wisdom and years of brainwashing tell us that this diet is indeed fundamentally unhealthy, but let's reconsider matters. It is true that Wolf did find many Rosetans to be overweight (though not by today's standards!). Perhaps this was to do with the regularity with which they ate sweet pastries by the time of his visits in the 1960s. But in spite of this, they had less heart disease and fewer heart attacks. Let's also remember that for the older Rosetans, the more frequent eating of sweet pastries was quite new and part of their gradual adaptation to American norms – a trend which was well underway by then. These long, healthy lives that Dr Wolf was examining were attributable to the sum total of what they had eaten and experienced throughout their lives – their diets

---

223 Gladwell, 2008, p.8.

and lifestyles dating back to the turn of the twentieth century or even earlier.

To start the process of reconsidering their dietary position, let's take a journey back to the early days of the Rosetan community soon after the founding of the township. A young priest, Father Pasquale de Nisco, took over at Our Lady of Mount Carmel in 1896. He played a major role in the community's development by importing and establishing

> 'Obsessed with the idea of the microbe, we often forget the most fundamental of all rules for the physician, that the right kind of food is the most important single factor in the promotion of health and the wrong kind of food the most important single factor in the promotion of disease.'
>
> *Dr Robert McCarrison… From his 1921 book* Studies in Deficiency Disease, *published at a time when knowledge of vitamins and their role in nutrition was slowly crystallising.*

their Italian way of life. He worked together with the townsfolk to clear the land and plant onions, beans, potatoes, melons and fruit trees including vines. As a result, in the words of the town's website today:[224] 'The town came to life. The Rosetans began raising pigs in their back yards, and growing grapes for homemade wine'. Life wasn't easy, but Roseto gradually morphed into a little slice of Italy embedded in the Pennsylvanian hills.

Right from the start of the twentieth century, the inhabitants of Roseto grew much of the food they ate and cooked it in their kitchens with a liberal use of lard. Dr Wolf documented with some distaste that:[225] 'They ate salami, hard and soft cheeses all brimming with cholesterol'. Yet now, with our feet firmly in the twenty-first century and the links between heart disease and high levels of dietary cholesterol having been disproven, perhaps Dr Wolf, were he alive today, would have commented differently. The American Heart Association changed their guidelines (back in the year 2000) and shifted their focus to saturated fat intake

---

224 www.boroughroseto.com/history
225 Bruhn and Wolf, 1979, Chapter 3: *The Rosetan Way of Life.*

rather than blood cholesterol which was, in any case, largely guilty by association. Simply because cholesterol can be found in most animal foods which also tend to be higher in saturated fat, it was seen as one of the 'heart attack' culprits. In January 2015, US Government guidelines were finally officially changed with the lifting of the longstanding caps on dietary cholesterol and the 'new' news that there was 'no appreciable relationship' between dietary cholesterol and blood cholesterol.[226] After nearly half a century of the needless avoidance of egg yolks, liver and shellfish, Americans were free to enjoy a broader and healthier diet again. There were, of course, no apologies for incorrect advice, or even for some of the damage which has been done. Nevertheless, these new guidelines are now gradually beginning to influence restaurant menus, school lunches and, of course, doctors' dieting advice. Tasteless egg-white omelettes should soon be a thing of the past! Just to put a final nail in that coffin, recent studies from countries as far apart as Norway and Taiwan support the growing research showing that low cholesterol levels are actually linked to higher rates of death for both men and women.[227]

When Wolf carried out his analysis, he automatically tagged the Rosetan diet as 'bad, and unhealthy'. To him, and to mainstream America, it was obvious that the standard American diet was better than what was on those dinner plates in Roseto, leading him to search elsewhere for answers to this paradox. But what about all this saturated fat they were eating in the form of lard, while mainstream America had virtually ditched the product by the mid-1960s? Was it really as heart-unhealthy as he believed?

Over the years, researchers and nutritionists have published many contradictory reports on the subject of how healthy saturated fats may or may not be. It's a complicated story. That being said, in a 1996 study of 43,757 health professionals,[228] the link between their saturated fat intake and their risk of heart disease was much weaker once the researchers took into consideration other factors such as their overall diet and fibre intake

---

226 United States Department of Agriculture, 2015.
227 Cheng et al., 2015; Nago et al., 2011.
228 Rimm et al., 1996.

(taking us back to the 'correlation not equalling causation' comment again). In a meta-analysis of 30,047 cases, 229 Dutch researchers reported that 'No evidence was found for an association between consumption of saturated fat and total cardiovascular disease.' And in a further meta-analysis comprising of 347,747 people published in 2010, researchers simply found insufficient evidence to link saturated fat to heart disease.[230]

Saturated fats have certainly been shown to be more benign than trans fats, which used to be found in margarine and vegetable shortening and were already a major constituent of our food intake by the middle of the twentieth century. During the early to middle part of the last century, Americans had converted to using foods rich in trans fatty acids such as Crisco shortening and omega-6 rich soy and cottonseed oils. The same process was happening, albeit more slowly, in other industrialised nations; cheaper margarine began to replace butter, and supposedly healthier cooking oils replaced beef tallow and lard. These days, trans fats are considered by most doctors to be the worst type of fat you can eat, but that was by no means the conventional wisdom at the time. Up until very recently, it was difficult to escape trans fats because for restaurants, they had almost magical qualities, providing nearly twice the usage of other oils and fats. Restaurants would use seed oils containing partially hydrogenated vegetable oil in their deep fryers, simply because they didn't have to change the oil as frequently. Although there are a few naturally occurring trans fats which are considered healthy, the commercially produced ones are manufactured in an industrial process that adds hydrogen to vegetable oil, making the oil solid at room temperature. So for trans fats, think solid oil.

It wasn't just the restaurants that loved trans fats. Food manufacturers loved their partially hydrogenated oils too because it made their candy bars and other processed foods less likely to spoil and gave them a longer shelf life. During the twentieth century we all got used to cooking and baking with more and more trans fats in our home kitchens too – and it all started with the launch of Crisco in the United States in 1911.

229 Hoenselaar, 2011.
230 Siri-Tarino et al., 2010.

Since the early 1800s, 'shortening' had been used as the generic term describing fats or oils which we added to baked goods to 'shorten' them or break up the gluten in flour, producing a more tender result. Biscuits such as shortbread are made lighter and flakier in spite of the sticky gluten content simply because of the added shortening, be it butter, lard or hydrogenated oil. Think Crisco if you're American; this was originally made from cottonseed oil, but these days consists of a blend of partially and fully hydrogenated soybean and palm oils. Think of brands such as Cookeen or Trex if you're British, Végétaline (made from hydrogenated coconut oil) if you're French, and Solo if you are from Belgium (where people still refer to margarine as baking butter or 'bakboter'). Wherever you live in the industrialised world, there will be a common brand name that was developed and sold as a solid oil created by this hydrogenation process.

So, by the 1950s and 1960s, the average American and many Europeans had dramatically changed their intake of fats and oils. Although trans fats are certainly edible, it is now acknowledged that eating them increases your risk of coronary heart disease; yet their consumption levels were already high across the United States in the 1950s and '60s – everywhere, it would seem, except in Roseto, where lard was king. They were spared the shift to Crisco in their kitchens – at least to some extent.

For the record: the use of trans fats is strictly controlled now within the European Union and in 2013, the American Food and Drugs Association decreed[231] that partially hydrogenated oils (which contain trans fats) are not 'generally recognised as safe'. This ruling was strengthened in 2015.

---

231 US Food and Drug Administration, 2015.

Some further observations on pork and lard

The lard the Rosetans used, the salami they made and the pork they ate came from their own locally pastured pigs. It was a far cry from the pork that most of us purchase today, which is sourced from industrial CAFOs (Concentrated Animal Feeding Operations) – these supply most of the pork we buy in supermarkets.

It is generally acknowledged that there are benefits associated with eating any animal raised in its natural habitat. With 'grass-fed' beef, we think of pasturing and green fields. But with pigs (and chickens too) it's different because they are natural omnivores; they literally eat a little bit of everything. So when it comes to pigs, just like chickens, terms such as 'free-range' are more accurate – but they stand for the same as grass-fed beef; namely, for a compassionate and ethical approach to raising animals.

Factory-farmed pigs trapped inside their CAFOs are fed largely on corn and soybean meal, often mixed with whatever else the agricultural industry needs to get rid of while still making them grow or gain weight quickly. Antibiotics are also an important part of their regular grub; interestingly (and rather disturbingly), an extraordinary 80% of all the antibiotics sold in the United States are fed to animals[232] – usually 'just in case'. The figure is so high at least partly because of the filthy and crowded conditions in which many animals find themselves.

With pork, the big issue is fat quality. This is, not surprisingly, directly related to their diet – which is pretty much anything they can get their snouts into! That covers roots, grass, leaves, grubs, nuts, berries, insects and more. If you choose to keep one in your back yard, as families often did in Europe during Victorian times (and many Rosetans used to), they will also be quite happy to eat up your table scraps. But the more grain there is in their diet, the higher their intake of omega-6 fats, and consequently, the higher the proportion of omega-6 in their meat

232 National Resources Defense Council, n.d.

and fat. One recent group of researchers[233] studied pigs whose diet was supplemented with 5% linseed oil (which is high in omega-3) while another group provided the control base. An analysis of the ham made at the end of the study showed a healthier ratio of 2.5:1 omega-6 fat to omega-3 compared to the control group with a ratio of 12:1.

We can safely assume that the omega-3 content of free-range Rosetan pigs was on the higher side, a fact which is today considered as making a positive contribution to human health.

Author's note: Interestingly, at my local Delhaize supermarket (near where I live in Belgium), although the pork sold there comes principally from factory farms, the labelling now clearly indicates that omega-3 supplements are added to the foodstuff they eat! To be fair, they also sell Iberian pork (at roughly twice the price), which comes from Spanish pigs whose diet includes large quantities of acorns and whose natural habitat means that they wander the fields and forests. Just for the record, it tastes great and is well worth the extra money. These days, I buy smaller portions of higher quality meat, or use the cheaper cuts for stews, so it's not actually costing me more.

---

233 Taranu et al., 2014.

Nutritional health

There are numerous other nutritional benefits associated with better quality meats and fats. Lard from pastured pigs is also rich in vitamin D, and (surprisingly to many) it is just like olive oil, classified as a mono-unsaturated fat. For comparison, lard is about 40% saturated, while butter is around 50%. From a food hygiene point of view, lard has a naturally long shelf life and does not go rancid quickly. With a high smoke point, lard represents one of the best fats for high-temperature cooking such as frying. Unlike many seed oils, lard is rich in saturated and mono-unsaturated fats considered 'stable', meaning that it does not form free radicals when heated.

Writing in *The Ecology of Disease:*

Medical opinion increasingly tends to accept that the food of industrial people is the most likely cause for the diseases of civilisation. But here again we encounter the sad fact of disagreement among scientists. If faulty food is the cause there is no agreement at all on what is the main fault. An excess of animal or saturated fat currently enjoys prominence as the main cause of our downfall, particularly as the cause of coronary heart disease, but evidence supporting this theory is not at all impressive.

Dr Walter Yellowlees, 1983 - Founder member of the McCarrison Society reaffirming the late Sir Robert McCarrison's belief that the most important factor in restoring health is healthy nutrition.

Poly-unsaturated corn and sunflower oils, for example, generate high levels of aldehydes when heated. These are known promoters of cancer, heart disease and dementia when eaten or inhaled. In a recent *BBC* documentary,[234] levels when frying were found to be twenty times higher than those recommended by the World Health Organisation.

---

234 *Trust Me, I'm a Doctor*, Could your cooking oils be damaging your health?, 2015.

In a recent *Washington Post* article,[235] the neuro-endocrinologist Thomas Sherman, Professor of Physiology at the Georgetown University Medical Center, urges his students to look at dietary choices – such as the decision to use lard – as a balancing act. He emphasises the right balance of carbohydrates to fats and proteins, and the right balance of the three kinds of fat. Apart from some other generally sound advice, Sherman advocates a diet with a variety of nutritious, minimally processed foods that are: 'reasonably low in sugars and carbs, rich in fruits and vegetables, and with a diversity of healthy fats that might well include some lard'. He also went on to say that: 'Lard isn't intrinsically good or bad. It's good if it's part of a healthy diet and bad if it's part of an unhealthy one. And if you have a good diet – a diet with a mix of different foods that's reasonably low in sugars and carbs, rich in fruits and vegetables, and has a diversity of healthy fats – I just don't see the harm in it'.

It is worth remembering that neither did the healthy citizens of Roseto all those years ago.

The US Dietary Guidelines Advisory Committee, which convenes every five years, is not yet convinced when it comes to the health benefits of saturated fats. But they have moderated their position, just as they did with cholesterol a few years back. The committee has now turned its core focus to added sugar, which is seen as the major villain for rising rates of obesity and type-2 diabetes. The gist of their 571-page-long report, published in early 2015,[236] was that egg yolks are back in fashion, that drinking coffee isn't bad, that moderate alcohol consumption is fine for you, as too are low amounts of saturated fat.

'There is a striking excess of added sugar intake in all age groups across the population,' commented Dr Krauss,[237] Director of Atherosclerosis Research at the Children's Hospital Oakland Research Institute and a former chairman of the American Heart Association's dietary guidelines committee. He went on to say that the advisory panel's emphasis on overall dietary patterns was: 'a tremendous move in the right direction'. As part of that move, the panel also quietly dropped its recommendation

---

235 Telis, 2013.
236 United States Department of Agriculture, 2015.
237 O'Connor, 2015.

from the previous guidelines that Americans restrict their total fat intake to 35 % of their daily calories.

My learning journey

By this time in my studies, I was coming round to the idea that fat was probably doing me more good than I had been led to believe – but only if it was the right kind. Picturing a simple set of scales, the benefits of fat were certainly outweighing those of the processed carbs (found in such things as sliced bread and chocolate pastries) on the other side of the balance. But I was trying to keep my mind open, while still reading the writings of Gary Taubes,[238] the science journalist, and Nina Teicholz,[239] the investigative journalist. They helped open my eyes to the full scale of intrigue around fat and cholesterol and their supposed links to an unhealthy diet.

> **The plaque-riddled state of American arteries was:**
>
> *'... dominated by the long- time effects of a rich fatty diet, and innumerable fat-loading meals'.*
>
> *Ancel Keys in 1957.*

The book that did most to influence me and remind me to really keep my eyes wide open was Denise Minger's *Death by Food Pyramid*.[240] If you read just one book on the history of how we ended up with today's poor nutritional guidelines and effectively in the hands of the processed food industry, this should be it. Don't worry; I am not a conspiracy theorist. There was no (and is no) master plan and no deliberate attempt to manipulate the situation into the hands of the greedy likes of Nestlé, Kraft and Kellogg's. But what the French describe as a 'concours de circonstances' came about, largely in the 1960s and '70s, and we find ourselves living the confusing end-result of those manoeuvres today. The book is a comparatively easy read, not telling you what to eat, but outlining from the author's point of view that we are all different, and that as a consequence, our dietary needs and wishes do not need to

238 Taubes, 2008.
239 Teicholz, 2014.
240 Minger, 2014.

be the same. She covers how politics and money ended up overriding the real scientific evidence before introducing us to two of the major protagonists: the American, Ancel Keys[241] (fat is bad) and the Englishman, John Yudkin (sugar is the real problem). These two figures are featured in a refreshingly even-handed way. Regarding dietary approaches such as Mediterranean, vegetarian and paleo, she notes that they all reduce processed and refined foods, sugars, trans fats and poly-unsaturated oils (such as seed oils). Could that be a clue in which direction we are headed?

---

241 The Ancel Keys quote in the text box above is from Teicholz, 2014, p.30.

How did the US government committees get diet recommendations so wrong?

The American investigative journalist, Nina Teicholz, spent ten years researching these fat- and cholesterol-based dietary issues before bringing out her book, *Big Fat Surprise*, in 2014. A recent *New York Times* article features her explaining the current 'scientific' situation:[242] 'The primary problem is that nutrition policy has long relied on a very weak kind of science: epidemiological or 'observational' studies in which researchers follow large groups of people over many years. But even the most rigorous epidemiological studies suffer from a fundamental limitation. At best they can show only association, not causation. Epidemiological data can be used to suggest hypotheses but not to prove them. Instead of accepting that this evidence was inadequate to give sound advice, strong-willed scientists overstated the significance of their studies'.

Teicholz has more recently added fuel to the fire by penning a well-read article for the *BMJ*[243] posing the following question: Why does the expert advice underpinning US government dietary guidelines not take account of all the relevant scientific evidence? In doing so, she has received much criticism from the established scientific community – yet the *BMJ* has taken a strong stance, declaring that they have:[244] '... also found that the committee's report used weak scientific standards'.

Yes indeed; the big-ego scientists with the loudest voices have usually won out. You'll have read the line 'correlation does not necessarily equal causation' several times in this book. Yet, as Teicholz says, many of the scientists who over the years have sought out evidence to support their theories have relied on this kind of statistical research (known as epidemiological). Such statistical inference only takes you so far, though, and if we'd had a few more scientists asking the question, 'What's really

---

242 Teicholz, 2015 (1).
243 Teicholz, 2015 (2).
244 Nestle, 2015.

going on?' rather than relying on the scientists who were following their hunches, we might find ourselves in a healthier place today. As it was, the outgoing and extroverted American food and diet scientist Ancel Keys – who followed his own 'hunches' about eating fat – is generally considered to have played the lead role in leading us onwards to the anti-cholesterol and low-fat era through which we are now living. He first presented his diet-fat-heart disease hypothesis (using the more technical word 'lipid' for fat) on an international stage at a 1955 meeting of the World Health Organization in Geneva, with, in the words of one observer, 'his usual confidence and bluntness'.[245]

Admittedly, at a later date, Ancel Keys went on to rescind his opinions on dietary cholesterol. But for those government bodies giving guidance and also for the press, cholesterol and fat were destined to be damned together as the principal causes of heart disease. The American public was surely also influenced by the reporting of President Eisenhower's heart attack in September of that same year, 1955. Just one day after the event (which the President survived), in an informatory press conference, his cardiologist, Dr Paul Dudley White, brought Americans up to speed on the causes of heart attacks, and also gave the following preventative advice:[246] 'Stop smoking, reduce stress, and on the dietary front, cut down on saturated fat and cholesterol'. It's worth noting that although Dwight Eisenhower had stopped smoking in 1951, he had, until then, smoked four packs a day for many years.

The inhabitants of Roseto in 1966 probably knew very little about Ancel Keys, but his message about fats and cholesterol was already becoming broadly

> **REMINDER**
> 'A reliable way to make people believe in falsehoods is frequent repetition, because familiarity is not easily distinguished from truth.
> Authoritarian institutions and marketers have always known this fact.'
>
> *Daniel Kahneman,* Thinking, Fast and Slow, *2011.*

---

245 Yerushalmy and Hilleboe, 1957.
246 In The New York Times, 26th September 1955 (quoted by Teicholz, 2014).

accepted in medical circles. Following his visits to Mediterranean countries, Ancel Keys was also becoming convinced that olive oil represented a healthier option, particularly when compared to cooking with animal fats, and he began communicating this in journals and during public speaking engagements. Given that background, when Dr Wolf's team saw the Rosetans still using lard, they (not surprisingly) jumped straight to the wrong conclusion, putting it down to the fact that the poor immigrants couldn't afford to import olive oil from their homeland to cook with. They didn't even consider that cooking with lard was an important part of their ancestral Italian cooking tradition; in fact, you will still find lard used extensively in Italy to this day. Interestingly, the finest lard in the world is still produced in Italy, and is eaten rather like salami. It fetches high prices, rather like Parma ham.

In the province of Puglia (where the original town of Roseto can be visited) located in the deep South East of Italy, the inhabitants enjoy one of the highest levels of life expectancy in the world. You will perhaps remember from an earlier chapter that Italy as a country comes tenth in the global life expectancy statistics, compared to the United States, which finds itself in place fifty-three.[247] When the original Rosetans left Italy for the United States towards the end of the nineteenth century, olive oil was sometimes used as a salad dressing but not frequently used for cooking. Although the olive oil marketing board has done a good job of positioning olive oil as a cooking ingredient with a long history, most olive oil production went towards heating and providing lamp light in the nineteenth century – just as beef tallow (fat) was used extensively for candles in other countries (read more on age 210). For thousands of years before then, olives were grown primarily to provide lamp oil, with little regard for culinary flavour. The advent of electricity changed all that, and new uses had to be found. Odysseus may well be famously quoted as using olive oil in *The Iliad*, but in reality, his personal usage most likely took the form of enhanced skincare; his food would have been cooked primarily using beef tallow and lard.

---

247 Geoba.se, 2015.

Yet in one sense, maybe it's good that Dr Wolf's focus was on community spirit and all that it represented. His research led him to the now well-documented conclusion that Roseto was an outlier to the rest of the United States because of the strong values they placed in family and community. He noted in particular that up to three generations in a family would live under one roof and that they willingly chose to live humble and simple lives.

This has anchored sociologists and psychologists in their opinion that social aspects of family, community and also simplicity of lifestyle lead to lower stress levels and happier people. And why not? It seems to me that leading simple lives and enjoying the community of family and friends have just as much to do with wellbeing as do eating a diet of real food and using fresh ingredients – perhaps a diet that's rich in animal fats, too? For the one thing that was clearly different about daily life in Roseto in the first half of the twentieth century (and to a lesser extent in the 1960s) was the relative absence of processed foods, the preference for locally produced vegetables and the use of locally sourced livestock. But that was all about to change.

Roseto re-joins the twentieth century

As Dr Wolf and his colleagues continued to monitor the health of the community, they noted that social change in the village was accompanied by increasing health problems. It was in 1971 that the very first heart attack death of a person aged less than forty-five occurred in Roseto.

Importantly, towards the end of the twentieth century, America's vulnerability to heart attacks and strokes began to decrease. This is attributed to many things, including the widespread adoption of exercise programmes, fewer people smoking, supposedly healthier diets and a big increase in the prescription of pills to reduce hypertension.

During the same time period, the Rosetans' comparative rates of heart disease steadily rose to match the national average; they effectively re-joined the rest of the United States. Like other mythical places, the older, healthier Roseto that used to exist in Pennsylvania has left us for the mists of scientific history. I would suggest, however, that many of the elements that made the town unique can still be found in the original Roseto, nestling in the Puglian hills. My subsequent visit there anchored me in my belief that their traditional cooking ingredients and methods certainly played a big role – together with their relatively fatty diet!

But the question still niggling me was really the following: could the demise of Roseto have been entirely down to the loss of a socially tight-knit community and all its benefits? It is true that young Rosetans today seldom stick around past childhood. However, in Dr Wolf's twenty-five-year review, published in 1990, he added a number of interesting annotations – including the fact that the inhabitants of Roseto had begun to consume less animal fat and more 'vegetable oils' (but not olive oil). I would put money on the fact that a closer look at the Rosetan diet of today would reveal very close similarities to the standard American diet (processed foods full of carbs and sugar and a high proportion of 'vegetable' oil extracted from seeds), in stark contrast to the more traditional and robust ways of cooking and eating that were enjoyed during the first half of the previous century.

Malcolm Gladwell is not the first to simply go along with today's conventional wisdom that saturated fats such as lard play an important role in a supposedly artery-clogging diet. In their best-selling book on communications, *Made to Stick*[248] (which came out around the same time as Gladwell's *Outliers: The Story of Success*), the Heath brothers delight in telling of the communicative powers of the then Head of the American Centre for Science in the Public Interest (CSPI), Art Silverman, and how, in 1994, he persuaded cinemas across the United States to drop the use of coconut oil (also a saturated fat because it's not liquid at room temperature) in their popcorn. You can imagine the scare it caused at the time when he declared that:[249] 'a large unbuttered popcorn had the saturated fat equivalent of six Big Macs'.

Saturated fat had been so demonised by then that when this mythology was combined with Art Silverman's convincing communication skills, the poor coconut oil suppliers had no chance! Now, I'm not personally advocating the consumption of popcorn at all, but sadly what replaced coconut oil was a retrograde step; cinemas began to use omega-6 rich soy and corn oil or maybe canola, each of them containing at the time alarmingly high levels of hydrogenated trans fats (subsequently reduced by law). To misquote Samuel Johnson: Art Silverman's good intentions took us somewhere along the pathway to hell.

And, for the record, coconut oil has now largely been redeemed. Today, it is most often used by health conscious paleo dieters and low-carb advocates.

---

248 Heath and Heath, 2007.
249 Heath and Heath, 2007, p.6.

Was my hunch correct? Could I prove it?

My hunch at this stage was that the use of lard from free-range pigs and the consumption of fresh vegetables and full-fat dairy produce, together with certain old-fashioned cooking methods employed by the Rosetans, played a major role in their good health. I wanted to find out whether we can still learn from them today. If fat is indeed good for us, I also wanted to find out what happens when your fat levels are at or above their reported 41%, and what adjustments need to be made to those other dietary constituents – primarily, the proportions of protein and carbohydrate that you should eat. Did the fact that they skipped the early part of the packaged and processed food revolution give them a twenty to thirty year advantage over the rest of us – in spite of the reported high levels of smoking? Could their fatty diet have been protective?

Another way of looking at this was to question whether the dominant dietary message of recent decades, namely 'eat low-fat foods and don't eat cholesterol-rich foods', should be giving way to a new regime, a new mantra. Perhaps it is 'consume more healthy fats and reduce your intake of processed foods'? I proceeded with my investigation ...

Why did Rosetans avoid heart disease for so long?

You can assess the quality of your health in many ways, with a general feel-good factor probably being top of the list on a day-to-day basis – particularly as you age. What we do know is that the Rosetans who lived through to the 1960s lived long, healthy lives and were not dying of heart disease; and yet now, they do ... just like everyone else. We all have to die of something, after all, but if we knew clearly and concisely why people get heart attacks, we could try and correlate that information to the habits of the Rosetans – at least as they used to be. We could gather clues to indicate if their long and healthy lives were really due to the benefits of living in their socially advantaged community – their little-Italy, in the heart of Pennysylvania.

If we had insights into why people suffer heart attacks, would it be possible to take a look and see what has changed over the years? As far as Roseto is concerned, we could benefit from the reports put together by Dr Wolf and his team of investigators for much of the necessary data. But a proportion of our considerations would simply have to be based on what we know generally about the lifestyle of the Rosetans – which hardly adds up to a true scientific study, I know. But perhaps such information might

> **What is cholesterol, anyway?**
> It's a waxy substance (a lipid) produced by the liver and found in certain foods; useful because it makes vitamin D, certain hormones, builds cell walls, and creates bile salts that help you digest fat. Your liver produces about one gram of cholesterol each day, and a quarter of the cholesterol in your body can be found in your brain.
>
> Makes you think!
>
> *Interestingly, among elderly people, the best memory function has been observed in those with the highest levels of cholesterol.*

provide us with additional reasons as to why these Italian Americans aged so gracefully – and maybe what we can still learn from them today.

To my pleasant surprise, it turns out that research in this area of medicine is a lot more solid than most of the nutrition research data that I have examined over the last few years. As long ago as 2004, a major and well-respected Canadian-led global study[250] identified nine easily measured risk factors that account for over 90% of heart attacks (or, as they called them, acute myocardial infarction). They were (and are):

1. Lipids (not absolute cholesterol levels, but measuring essentially the ratio of HDL (good) to LDL (bad) cholesterol).

2. Smoking.

3. Diabetes.

4. Hypertension.

5. Obesity.

6. Psychosocial factors (stress).

These six factors were found to represent over 80% of the risk associations. Adding to that, diet, physical activity and moderate alcohol consumption were shown to have the opposite effect; namely, they have been shown to exert a positive influence on your total heart-attack risk. With this list of just nine variables, the researchers were able to identify over 90% of all heart-attack risk factors.

The study, named 'Interheart', showed (equally surprisingly) that these nine risk factors are the same all around the world; that they affect every racial and ethnic group and that they are valid for both men and women. And this was a sizeable study, positively reviewed by peer groups. They matched over fifteen thousand people who had experienced at least one heart attack with fifteen thousand who had no history of heart disease.

---

250 Brooks, 2004.

Currently, death rates from coronary heart disease vary greatly around the world. For men, the figures range from 35 per 100,000 in South Korea to 733 in the Ukraine. For women, they range from a low rate of 11 in France to 313 – again in the Ukraine.[251] But, independent of those figures, the risk factors remain the same.

Taking a brief look at the Interheart risk factors:

1. A major risk factor was **Lipids** – rather than using total cholesterol levels as the key risk indicator (which most early researchers had done), this study used the 'consistent and independent' relationship between elevated ApoB/ApoA to identify risk; ApoB being the major protein in LDL Lipoproteins and ApoA being the major protein in HDL particles. (***Lipids are substances containing fats*** such as fatty acids, oils, waxes, sterols, and triglycerides – and, of course, cholesterol.)

2. No surprise here: **Smoking** – just 1–5 cigarettes smoked daily increases your risk by 38%, but with higher daily levels, the figures sky-rocket.

3. **Hypertension** – an important factor which may have been underestimated, since this factor was self-reported.

4. **Diabetes** – this also may have been underestimated, since this factor was self-reported.

5. **Obesity** – interestingly, abdominal obesity (waist size) proved to be a greater risk factor than BMI (Body Mass Index).

6. **Psychosocial factors** (stress) – including stress at work or home, financial stress, stressful life events, depression and the perceived ability to control your life circumstances ... not to be underestimated!

---

251 Nowbar et al., 2014.

These six factors represented over 80% of the risk associations. On the potentially positive side were:

7. Diet – the study only controlled for whether you eat fruit and veg on a daily basis, yet this certainly proved to be a protective factor.

8. Physical activity – both moderate (walking, for example) and strenuous exercise were seen as being protective.

9. Alcohol – a protective effect was seen with moderate alcohol consumption, balanced against the potential health risks of excessive use.

These three potentially positive categories brought the total predictive risk factors up to just above 90%, so a review to see how Roseto measures up against these criteria could be a great starting point.

To our modern ears, there are probably no major surprises in this list. But in the medical world, the results were seen as being so conclusive that they really became quite a big deal.

In the words of Dr Jean-Pierre Després of the Quebec Heart Institute when speaking at the ESC conference where this study was first presented:[252] 'We have to reshape our working and living environments and address cultural and social factors favouring destructive behaviours'. He added the warning that: '… mankind is doing a good job of killing itself'.

Now, let's go back to Roseto and see how they measured up against these risk factors – both at the time of the original work in the early 1960s and twenty-five years later on when Dr Wolf wrote his updated report. We must remember that the number of Rosetans in the survey who had experienced one or more myocardial infarctions in 1985 was more than double the 1960s figure.

---

252 As reported by Brooks, 2004.

	Rosetans – 1960s	Twenty-five years on (Dr Wolf's 1988 report)
Cholesterol	High.	'There was not a significant change in blood cholesterol concentration among Rosetans over the 25 year span.'
HDL to LDL	Probably high (at the time, only total cholesterol was considered relevant).	No specific measurements or comments.
Smoking	Yes.	'In 1985 we found a decrease in the number of Rosetans who smoked. The decrease was evident only among the men, however.'
Diabetes	Low – no differences to other local communities.	No specific measurements or comments.
Hypertension	No information.	'… the prevalence of hypertension had increased sharply in Roseto over the 25 year interval.'
Obesity	Some reported as being 'overweight' at the time.	No additional comments.
Psychosocial (benefits of a close-knit community)	They experienced many of the same social problems and personal conflicts as their neighbours, but had a philosophy of cohesion with powerful support from family and deep religious convictions. Additionally, mental illness (including dementia) was much lower: half the rate of Bangor, and only a third the rate of Nazareth.	Dwindling community values as Roseto became more typical of other American towns. More social interaction with other communities; increased signs of ostentation, particularly among younger Rosetans. No further comments on mental health.

Diet	Fewer processed foods; many fresh vegetables; diet high in 'saturated fat & cholesterol'.	'The individual data on dietary habits indicated a clear but modest decrease in the consumption of salt, animal fat and lard, and more use of corn oil in cooking. Consumption of olive oil among Rosetans was less than that of other oils in 1985, just as it had been in 1963.'… whatever dietary changes had occurred in our 25 year follow-up had been in the direction of what the AMA calls 'prudent' – less consumption of animal fat, less smoking and less exercise.'
Alcohol	Considered to be on the high side.	There was relatively little change in drinking habits among Rosetans during the 25 year interval except for a moderate reduction in hard liquor consumption.
Physical Exercise	Considered to be moderate (more so for those men still working in the slate mines). Lots of social walking.	The long-standing tradition of Rosetans walking about the town in the evening visiting with neighbours began to fade and by 1985 was hardly observed at all. By 1985 many fewer Rosetans were engaged in labouring jobs than in the 1960s. Those who formerly walked to the neighbourhood stores for groceries, goods and services began to drive to the supermarkets elsewhere.

What can we ascertain from all this?

With no significant differences when it comes to the reported levels of smoking and drinking alcohol, little information relating to diabetes and just some mentions of being overweight (but no reported cases of obesity), we are left with the following:

The town of Roseto lost its heart-protective aura and levels of hypertension increased sharply during a time in which the following happened:

- The cohesive nature of their shared community values dwindled.

- They reduced their levels of casual exercise and movement (i.e. walking), adopting a more sedentary lifestyle.

- Their diet became 'Westernised'.

The contemporary sociologist's analysis has focused on the loss of shared community and family values, but could those psychological aspects alone have been enough to bring about such a major change in their rates of heart disease?

What about the exercise factor? We are learning today that gentle exercise is just as important as going to the gym when it comes to leading longer, healthier lives. As Dr Wolf reported twenty-five years on:[253] '... the long-standing tradition of Rosetans walking about the town in the evening visiting with neighbors began to fade and by 1985 was hardly observed at all. Those who formerly walked to the neighborhood stores for groceries, goods and services, began to drive to the supermarkets elsewhere'.

The degree to which this may have reduced the total level of exercise for Rosetans is difficult to estimate – but when combined with the reduction in number of Rosetans engaged in labouring jobs compared to the 1960s, it is certainly noteworthy.

---

253 Wolf et al., 1989, p.66.

When it came to their cooking and eating habits at the time of the first analysis, now over fifty years ago, their diet was seen as yet another negative factor to be equated with high levels of smoking. Just listen to Dr Wolf:[254] 'I've had many dinners with Rosetan families. They usually have more than one type of meat. When I eat ham I cut the rim of fat off and don't eat it, same way with roast beef, but they cut right through and eat it all. We were very elaborate in our study of their diet because we had Ancel Keys breathing down our necks'.

In his '25 years later' report, Dr Wolf related further stories from earlier days with Rosetan families:[255] 'The oil intake of the Rosetans was relatively low in olive oil. They used a great deal more lard than the wives of the people in this room use. One of their favorite dishes was fried peppers. They would fry the peppers in lard and they are very good. Then you'd take a piece of Italian bread and rub it around in the gravy that is left and eat that, and that's delicious!'.

In the 1960s, with America moving fast in the 'healthy low-fat, low cholesterol' direction, it's not surprising how Dr Wolf and his contemporaries looked at these 'unhealthy' eating habits. It is only with today's eyes that we can again begin to consider whether eating saturated fats such as butter and lard may be a good thing in comparison to the 'vegetable' oils from maize, soy, sunflower etc. When put in the dietary context of the fresh local vegetables they grew, an absence of pre-packaged, processed and fast food and locally sourced free-range meat, it seems increasingly likely that their diet actually had a protective effect on their hearts.

---

254 Wolf et al., 1989, p.67.
255 Idem.

All things change

Dr Wolf's study of Roseto was originally prompted by a comment from a local physician, Dr Benjamin Falcone, who had been practising there for seventeen years. He made it to Stewart Wolf in 1961, the year President Kennedy was elected, declaring that he rarely saw a case of myocardial infarction in any of the 1,600 inhabitants of Roseto under the age of sixty-five. Later, after studying the people and the data, Dr Wolf went on record as saying:[256] 'In 1963, we boldly made and recorded a prediction that, should the inhabitants of Roseto abandon their traditional values and behavior, they would lose their relative immunity from fatal myocardial infarction'.

I certainly don't want to downplay the tremendous changes to their traditions and their sense of community which were sadly fading away as Roseto caught up with the modern world; they were playing catch-up, after all. Those changes were seen in many ways, as the following quotes illustrate:[257]

'Their community pride and group morale appeared to have been partially displaced by concern with personal status and power.'

'The number of three generation households had diminished greatly. Between 1960 and 1980 the population of Roseto had decreased by 8% but the number of households had increased by the same percentage.'

'Elderly Rosetans, previously cared for at home, had been entered into nursing homes.'

'People joined country clubs and attendance at the men's clubs in Roseto declined. There was even a decline in church attendance at the local Catholic Church. Marriages, which had traditionally been to Italians, were becoming ethnically mixed.'

But the thing is, they were not simply in the process of changing their social interactions and adopting new 'modern' social infrastructures; they

---

256 Idem, p.63.
257 Idem, pp. 60 – 62.

were making fundamental changes to their lifestyles and diet – catching up with a process of Americanisation which had started phasing-in to the younger members of their society already in the late 1950s.

I am not the first to raise the question of the positive role their diet might have played. Ancel Keys himself reviewed the data but dismissed the dietary comments in the original report as 'an aberration' since it certainly did nothing to support his 'fat is bad for your heart' theory.[258] A different diet-related viewpoint came from the founder (Dr Fishman, writing under her *nom de plume*, Aldebaran) of a society named *Fat Underground* which supported portly people in the USA. Fishman noted that the Rosetans were not the slimmest of folk, and wrote the following paragraph in the *Los Angeles Times* on January 6th, 1976: 'These Rosetans are notably fat as a group and cheerfully consume large quantities of high-calorie, high-cholesterol Italian foods. Yet they enjoy remarkably good general health, dying from heart disease at about one-third of the national toll, and being afflicted with diabetes at only a quarter of the rate of the population at large'.[259]

If their diet did play a positive role in creating their healthy hearts, that information is highly relevant to society today. Funnily enough, that diet of theirs was based to a great extent on the Mediterranean diet still prevalent today back 'home' in the Puglian region of Southern Italy. But that genuine Mediterranean diet only has certain things in common with the much-touted olive oil and oily fish version which does the rounds today. Olive oil and fish are surely good for you, but just as important may be freshly grown local vegetables, unleavened or sourdough breads made from local durum wheat and farm-raised meat and animal fats in the form of lard and butter. Their enhanced sense of community certainly played a role too, and being a bit overweight doesn't seem to have harmed them either – so perhaps Western society's fixation on the perfect dream figure provides a further stumbling block for our healthy aspirations today.

---

258 Keys, 1966.
259 As reported by Szwarc, 2008.

Conclusion

Today's epidemics of diabetes and obesity are certainly interlinked and being a little fat in those 1960's terms has little to do with today's highly enhanced waistlines fuelled by junk food and in particular, cheap refined carbohydrates. We must first learn again how to eat right and in so doing, we will begin to tackle the more serious issue of obesity, just as Katy learned to do. The low-fat experiment which various food and government authorities have imposed on us for these past 40 years or so has failed disastrously. Combined with the ill-fated and misguided use of calories to measure and control our weight, this massive experiment with Western society has resulted in having precisely the opposite effect to that intended. The repeated mass communication that fat, especially animal fat, will do you harm has worked to the point that people today feel guilty when making simple buying decisions such as choosing whole fat over low-fat milk. In the United States, which has led the way in using many differing communications channels for this message of indoctrination; sales of whole fat milk decreased by 61 per cent, sales of 2% milk increased by 106 per cent and sales of 1% and skimmed milk increased by over 160 per cent, between 1975 and 2014.[260]

It is time to accept that we have been successfully brainwashed to the point that most of us still choose the reduced fat option and think we are doing the right thing. Only when we begin to lose our fear of fat and embrace healthy fats in our diet will we regain the ability to restore health, reduce diseases such as type-2 diabetes that are largely of our own making and start work on reducing our expanding waistlines.

---

260 USDA statistics quoted in Messinger, 2015.

ADDENDUM

Since completing this book at the end of 2015, the 2016-20 American Dietary Guidelines have been published. Although these guidelines only affect us indirectly in Europe, they tend to lead the way for our everyday conventional thinking when it comes to food and diet. This is partly because of the enormous soft-power of American media and partly because so many US-based food multinationals adjust their processed foods recipes and develop new marketing ideas aligned to the new opportunities presented by such updated guidelines.

Admittedly, there are no major changes this time around, other than limits being removed from what we should eat when it comes to those foods containing cholesterol. Eggs are officially OK again (hurrah) – and by the by, it is also good to see fewer mentions of low-fat foods in the new guidelines.

The whole thought process, though, is still very much driven by counting calories. Refreshing as it may be to read that sugar intake should now be restricted to less than 10% of those daily calories, that same 10% measure is also applied to your daily ration of saturated fats, be they from milk, butter or coconut oil. As you will understand, as far as I am concerned, this new guidance fails to address today's most pressing issues.

Until our 'government-guideline-fed' phobia of fat goes away, we will not begin to eat enough natural, real foods and we will continue searching for processed goods that are developed and segmented in line with these written criteria. It does not take a clairvoyant to see that as 2016 rolls out, new butter-like spreads will doubtless emerge with phrases like 'healthier, with no saturated fat' or '0% sat fat' just as the 'no-cholesterol' banners emerged in earlier years. Such new product lines will emerge in the USA and cross the pond to reach British supermarkets a little later. By 2017, we'll be seeing them 'on the continent'.

Looking on the bright side, those scientists advising the government have made a massive shift away from condemning all fats and putting them in the 'bad for your health' category. But – and it's a big but – they have not shown themselves to be brave enough to tackle the broader category of highly processed junk food which contains the starches and sugars that are fuelling our poor eating habits, our declining health and our expanding waistlines.

TABLE OF FIGURES

Figure 1: 1941 Poster. Should you eat like your great-grandma? Looks quite healthy, don't you think?
(Source: photograph of an old US Govt poster)

Figure 2: The original US Food Guide Pyramid
(Source: http://www.nal.usda.gov/fnic/Fpyr/pyramid.gif)

Figure 3: ... morphed into the 'eatwell plate' (NHS, UK). Fat and sugar are still lumped together in the smallest section!
(Source: https://www.gov.uk/government/publications/the-eatwell-plate-how-to-use-it-in-promotional-material/the-eatwell-plate-how-to-use-it-in-promotional-material)

Figure 4: Is obese becoming the new normal?
(Source: author's own)

Figure 5: Looks good ... but toast, fried potatoes, beans and carb-rich sausages are to be avoided.
(Source: author's own)

Figure 6: Still a fine, filling breakfast; just make sure the sausages are at least 90% meat to ensure a delicious low-carb start to the day.
(Source: author's own)

Figure 7: From Measuring Up – a 2013 report on the UK's obesity crisis.
(Source: The State of Food and Agriculture 2013. United Nations Food and Agricultural Organization http://www.fao.org/docrep/018/i3300e/i3300e.pdf. Easy view at: www.nhs.uk/Livewell/loseweight/Pages/statistics-and-causes-of-the-obesity-epidemic-in-the-UK.aspx)

Figure 8: Daniel Lambert weighed 50 stone (over 300 kilos) at the time of his death in 1809. He charged people money to see him in shows; a sign of how rare obesity used to be.
(Sources: Wikipedia (entry for Daniel Lambert); 'Marshall Lambert' by Benjamin Marshall - Dictionary of National Biography. Original, Leicestershire Museums and Art Galleries. Licensed under Public Domain via Commons -https://commons.wikimedia.org/wiki/File:Marshall_Lambert.jpg#/media/File:Marshall_Lambert.jpg)

Figure 9: New York dancer, 1890 – this plumper body ideal was soon to change. (Source: Charles McCaghy collection at Ohio State University – public domain; http://hdl.handle.net/1811/47626)

Figure 10: Burlesque dancer, Mlle Conalba – not the physique of today's dancers. (Source: Charles McCaghy collection at Ohio State University – public domain; http://hdl.handle.net/1811/47663)

Figure 11: The flappers helped change women's role in society – and promoted a skinnier physique.
(Source: public domain; widely used)

Figure 12: The body, seen as a food-burning furnace – from Diet and Health by Dr Hunt-Peters, 1918.
(Source: 'Lulu Peters Diet and Health, 1918, p13' by Chemical Heritage Foundation. Licensed under Public Domain via Commons - https://commons.wikimedia.org/wiki/File:Lulu_Peters_Diet_and_Health_1918_p13.jpg#/media/File:Lulu_Peters_Diet_and_Health_1918_p13.jpg)

Figure 13: Please note the lack of similarity between a bomb calorimeter and the human digestive system.
(Source: public domain)

Figure 14: Billy Bunter – the 1950s TV star as portrayed by Gerald Campion. (Source: BBC Television)

Figure 15: Just one of these cream doughnuts contains 51 grams of carbs, 27 grams of which is sugar.
(Source: author's own)

Figure 16: UK sugar consumption figures 1700-1978, with US figures for 1975-2000 added in black. Compare with obesity rates in US for those aged 60-69.
(Source: author's own, derived from: UK sugar consumption figures 1700-1978 in Johnson et al., 2007. Potential role of sugar (fructose) in the epidemic of hypertension, obesity and the metabolic syndrome, diabetes, kidney disease, and cardiovascular disease. American Journal of Clinical Nutrition: http://ajcn.nutrition.org/content/86/4/899.full.pdf+html)

Figure 17: If someone were to create a drug as effective as the slow-burning nature of eating fat ...
(Source: author's own)

Figure 18: Carbohydrates are the main ingredients in junk food.
(Source: iStock.com/Goce)

Figure 19: These figures show the impact of improved children's health.
(Source: Extracts from A Century of Change: Trends in UK statistics since 1900)

Figure 20: Heart disease and cancer – the most common causes of death today.
(Source: Extracts from A Century of Change: Trends in UK statistics since 1900)

Figure 21: Troops of the 1900 Eight Nations Alliance. Left to right: Britain, USA, Australia, India, Germany, France, Russia, Italy and Japan.
(Source: 'Troops of the Eight nations alliance 1900' by Anonymous - Historica, Yamagawa shuppan. Licensed under Public Domain via Commons – https://commons.wikimedia.org/wiki/File:Troops_of_the_Eight_nations_alliance_1900.jpg#/media/File:Troops_of_the_Eight_nations_alliance_1900.jpg)

Figure 22: Yes – there really did used to be a British Lard Marketing Board. This ad is from 1958.
(Source: public domain)

Figure 23: Shop sign; photo taken at the Colonatta Lard Festival, every August in Tuscany.
(Source: author's own)

Figure 24: Omega-6 vs Omega-3 content in oils.
(Source: http://chriskresser.com/how-too-much-omega-6-and-not-enough-omega-3-is-making-us-sick)

REFERENCES

Accurso, A. et al. (2008) Dietary carbohydrate restriction in type 2 diabetes mellitus and metabolic syndrome: time for a critical appraisal. Nutrition and Metabolism. [Online] Available from: http://www.nutritionandmetabolism.com/content/5/1/9 [Accessed: 15th January 2016].

Allentoft, M. et al. (2015) Population genomics of Bronze Age Eurasia. Nature. [Online] Available from: http://www.nature.com/nature/journal/v522/n7555/full/nature14507.html [Accessed: 15th January 2016].

American Heart Association. (2000) An Eating Plan for Healthy Americans. [Online] Available from: http://www.med.navy.mil/sites/nhyoko/Documents/WellnessCenter/SelfHelpMaterials/AHA%20EATING%20PLAN.pdf [Accessed: 15th January 2016].

American Heart Association. (2015) Inflammation and Heart Disease. [Online] Available from: http://www.heart.org/HEARTORG/Conditions/Inflammation-and-Heart-Disease_UCM_432150_Article.jsp#.Vm0iZPkrKhc [Accessed: 15th January 2016].

American Liver Foundation. (2015) NAFLD. Non-Alcoholic Fatty Liver Disease. [Online] Available from: http://www.liverfoundation.org/abouttheliver/info/nafld/ [Accessed: 15th January 2016].

Atkins, R. (1972) Dr Atkins' Diet Revolution. Bantam Books.

Australian Heart Foundation. (n.d.) Waist measurement. [Online] Available from: http://heartfoundation.org.au/your-heart/know-your-risks/healthy-weight/waist-measurement [Accessed: 15th January 2016].

AverageHeight.co (n.d.) Average Male Height by Country. [Online] Available from: http://www.averageheight.co/average-male-height-by-country

Basaranoglu, M. et al. (2015) Carbohydrate intake and nonalcoholic fatty liver disease: fructose as a weapon of mass destruction. Hepatobiliary Surg Nutr. [Online] Apr; 4(2): 109–116. Available from: http://www.ncbi.nlm.nih.gov/pmc/articles/PMC4405421/ [Accessed: 15th January 2016].

Blair Johnson, N. et al. (2014) Leading Causes of Morbidity and Mortality and Associated Behavioral Risk and Protective Factors—United States, 2005–2013. Centers for Disease Control and Prevention MMWR [Online] 31st October. 63(04);3–27. Available from: http://www.cdc.gov/mmwr/preview/mmwrhtml/su6304a2.htm [Accessed: 15th January 2016].

Brookes, L. (2004) INTERHEART: A Global Case-Control Study of Risk Factors for Acute Myocardial Infarction. Medscape [Online] Available from: http://www.medscape.com/viewarticle/489738 [Accessed: 15th January 2016].

Brown, P. (2015) BMJ Lambasts U.S. Dietary Group for Shoddy Research - Article claims USDA guidelines are based on 'weak scientific standards'. Medpage Today. [Online] 24th September. Available from: http://www.medpagetoday.com/PrimaryCare/DietNutrition/53701 [Accessed: 15th January 2016].

Bruhn, J. G. and Wolf, S. (1979) The Roseto Story: An Anatomy of Health. Norman: University of Oklahoma.

Buettner, D. (2008) The Blue Zones: Lessons for Living Longer From the People Who've Lived the Longest. National Geographic Books.

Buettner, D. (2012) The Island Where People Forget to Die. The New York Times Magazine. [Online] 24th October. Available from: http://www.nytimes.com/2012/10/28/magazine/the-island-where-people-forget-to-die.html?_r=0 [Accessed: 15th January 2016].

Campbell, M. K. and Farrell, S. O. (2015) Biochemistry. 8th Ed. Cengage Learning.

Carnethon, M. R. et al. (2012) Association of Weight Status with Mortality in Adults with Incident Diabetes. The Journal of the American Medical Association. [Online] Aug 8; 308(6):581–90. Available from: http://jama.jamanetwork.com/article.aspx?articleid=1309174 [Accessed: 15th January 2016].

Carroll, A.E. (2015) No, You Do Not Have to Drink 8 Glasses of Water a Day. The New York Times. [Online] 24th August. Available from: http://www.nytimes.com/2015/08/25/upshot/no-you-do-not-have-to-drink-8-glasses-of-water-a-day.html?_r=1 [Accessed: 15th January 2016].

Castelli, W. P. (1992) Concerning the Possibility of a Nut.... Arch Intern Med. [Online] 152(7):1371–1372. Available from: http://archinte.jamanetwork.com/article.aspx?articleid=616375 [Accessed: 15th January 2016].

Cavan, D. (2014) Reverse your Diabetes: the step-by-step plan to take control of type 2 diabetes. London: Vermillion.

Chamsi-Pasha, H. (2015) Saturated fats: Good, Bad or Ugly? BMJ (Rapid Responses). [Online] 14th August. Available from: http://www.bmj.com/content/351/bmj.h3978?sort_by=field_highwire_a_epubdate_value&sort_order=DESC&items_per_page=10&page=1&panels_ajax_tab_tab=bmj_related_rapid_responses&panels_ajax_tab_trigger=rapid-responses [Accessed: 15th January 2016].

Cheng, K. H. et al. (2015) Lipid paradox in acute myocardial infarction – the association with 30-day in-hospital mortality. Crit Care Med. [Online]

Jun; 43(6):1255–64. Available from: http://www.ncbi.nlm.nih.gov/pubmed/25738856 [Accessed: 15th January 2016].

Choi, C. (2015) Coca-Cola paid nutrition experts to recommend soda as a healthy snack. Business Insider UK. [Online] 17th March. Available from: http://uk.businessinsider.com/coca-cola-paid-nutrition-experts-to-recommend-soda-as-a-healthy-snack-2015-3?r=US&IR=T [Accessed: 15th January 2016].

Chowdhury, R. et al. (2014) Association of Dietary, Circulating, and Supplement Fatty Acids With Coronary Risk. Annals of Internal Medicine. [Online] 18 March, Vol. 160. No. 6: 398–406. Available from: http://annals.org/article.aspx?articleid=1846638 [Accessed: 15th January 2016].

Cohen, S. et al. (2006) Positive Emotional Style Predicts Resistance to Illness After Experimental Exposure to Rhinovirus or Influenza A Virus. Psychosom Med. [Online] 2006 Nov–Dec; 68(6):809–15. Available from: http://repository.cmu.edu/cgi/viewcontent.cgi?article=1272&context=psychology [Accessed: 15th January 2016].

Colditz, G. A. (1991) Epidemiology of Breast Cancer. Findings from the Nurses' Health Study. Cancer. [Online] Volume 71, Issue Supplement S4. Available from: http://onlinelibrary.wiley.com/doi/10.1002/cncr.2820710413/pdf [Accessed: 15th January 2016].

Connor, T. (2014) Autoimmune Disease and The Paleo Diet: Case Studies. [Online] 27th February 2014. Available from: http://thepaleodiet.com/autoimmune-disease-and-the-paleo-diet-case-studies/ [Accessed: 15th January 2016].

Craig, C. (2015) A Ketogenic Diet For ME/CFS & Fibro [Online] 30th March 2015. Available from: http://www.drcourtneycraig.com/blog/2015/3/25/a-ketogenic-diet-for-mecfs-fibro [Accessed: 15th January 2016].

Credit Suisse Research Institute (2015) Fat: The New Health Paradigm. [Online] September 2015. Available from: http://publications.credit-suisse.com/tasks/render/file/index.cfm?fileid=9163B920-CAEF-91FB-EE5769786A03D76E [Accessed: 15th January 2016].

Crisp, N. (2010) Turning the World Upside Down: the search for global health in the 21st Century. London: Royal Society of Medicine Press.

Czeisler, C. A. (2006) Sleep deficit: the performance killer. A conversation with Harvard Medical School Professor Charles A. Czeisler. Harv Bus Rev. [Online] 2006 Oct;84(10):53–9, 148. Available from: http://www.ncbi.nlm.nih.gov/pubmed/17040040 [Accessed: 15th January 2016].

Daley, C. et al. (2010) A review of fatty acid profiles and antioxidant content in grass-fed and grain-fed beef. Nutr J. [Online] 2010; 9:10. Available from:

http://www.ncbi.nlm.nih.gov/pmc/articles/PMC2846864/ [Accessed: 15th January 2016].

David, A. R. and Zimmerman, M. R. (2010) Cancer: an old disease, a new disease or something in between? Nature Reviews Cancer [Online] 10, 728–733 (October 2010). Available from: http://www.nature.com/nrc/journal/v10/n10/abs/nrc2914.html [Accessed: 15th January 2016].

Dayton, S. et al. (1969) A Controlled Clinical Trial of a Diet High in Unsaturated Fat in Preventing Complications of Atherosclerosis. Circulation. [Online] 1969; 40: II-1-II-63. Available from: http://circ.ahajournals.org/content/40/1S2/II-1.short [Accessed: 15th January 2016].

de Souza, R. J. et al. (2015) Intake of saturated and trans unsaturated fatty acids and risk of all cause mortality, cardiovascular disease, and type 2 diabetes: systematic review and meta-analysis of observational studies. BMJ [Online] 2015; 351:h3978. Available from: http://www.bmj.com/content/351/bmj.h3978 [Accessed: 15th January 2016].

Diabetes UK. (n.d.) Pear and almond traybake. [Online] Available from: https://www.diabetes.org.uk/Guide-to-diabetes/Recipes/Pear-and-almond-traybake/ [Accessed: 15th January 2016].

Diamond, J. (1987) The Worst Mistake in the History of the Human Race. Discover Magazine. [Online] May 1987, pp. 64–66. Available from: http://www.ditext.com/diamond/mistake.html [Accessed: 15th January 2016].

Djousse, L. et al. (2010). Chocolate consumption is inversely associated with calcified atherosclerotic plaque in the coronary arteries: The NHLBI Family Heart Study. Clinical Nutrition [Online] 30 (2011) 38–43. Available from: http://www.sacredchocolate.com/docs/sacredpdf/chocolate-consumption-reverse-atherosclerotic-plaque.pdf [Accessed: 15th January 2016].

Dodson, E. R. and Zee, P. C. (2010) Therapeutics for Circadian Rhythm Sleep Disorders. Sleep Med Clin. [Online] 2010 Dec; 5(4):701–715. Available from: http://www.ncbi.nlm.nih.gov/pmc/articles/PMC3020104/ [Accessed: 15th January 2016].

Ebbeling, C. B. et al. (2012) Effects of dietary composition on energy expenditure during weight-loss maintenance. The Journal of the American Medical Association [Online] 2012 Jun 27;307(24):2627–34. Available from: http://jama.jamanetwork.com/article.aspx?articleid=1199154 [Accessed: 15th January 2016].

EFEMA. (2015) History. [Online] Available from: http://www.emulsifiers.org/ViewDocument.asp?ItemId=9 [Accessed: 15th January 2016].

Egolf, B. et al. (1992) The Roseto effect: a 50-year comparison of mortality rates. Am J Public Health. 1992 August; 82(8):1089–1092. [Online] Available from: http://www.ncbi.nlm.nih.gov/pmc/articles/PMC1695733/ [Accessed: 15th January 2016].

Elmore, B. J. (2015) Citizen Coke: The Making of Coca-Cola Capitalism. New York: W. W. Norton & Company.

Emsley, J. (2012) What's inside Flora Pro.Active Light. Wired. [Online] 7th March. Available from: http://www.wired.co.uk/magazine/archive/2012/04/start/whats-inside-flora-pro [Accessed: 15th January 2016].

Estruch, R. et al. (2013) Primary Prevention of Cardiovascular Disease with a Mediterranean Diet. N Engl J Med 2013; 368:1279-1290. [Online] Available from: http://www.nejm.org/doi/full/10.1056/NEJMoa1200303#t=articleTop [Accessed: 15th January 2016].

EUFIC. (2001) Gut microflora: the inside story. [Online] Available from: http://www.eufic.org/article/en/artid/gut-microflora/ [Accessed: 15th January 2016].

Fan, M. S. et al. (2008) Evidence of decreasing mineral density in wheat grain over the last 160 years. J Trace Elem Med Biol. [Online] 2008;22(4):315-24. Available from: http://www.ncbi.nlm.nih.gov/pubmed/19013359 [Accessed: 15th January 2016].

Feldman, S. and Marks, V. (2006) Panic Nation. London: John Blake Publishing Ltd.

Fields, S. (2004) The Fat of the Land: Do Agricultural Subsidies Foster Poor Health? Environ Health Perspect. [Online] 2004 Oct; 112(14): A820–A823. Available from: http://www.ncbi.nlm.nih.gov/pmc/articles/PMC1247588/ [Accessed: 15th January 2016].

First Do No Harm. (1997) Film. Directed by Jim Abrahams. [DVD] Walt Disney Video.

Forbes Magazine. (2007) World's Fattest Countries. [Online] Available from: http://www.forbes.com/2007/02/07/worlds-fattest-countries-forbeslife-cx_ls_0208worldfat.html [Accessed: 15th January 2016].

Foster, G. D. et al. (2010) Weight and metabolic outcomes after 2 years on a low-carbohydrate versus low-fat diet: a randomized trial. Ann Intern Med. [Online] 2010 Aug 3;153(3):147-57. Available from: http://www.ncbi.nlm.nih.gov/pubmed/20679559 [Accessed: 15th January 2016].

Framingham Heart Study. (n.d.) (1) About the Framingham Heart Study. [Online] Available from: https://www.framinghamheartstudy.org/about-fhs/ [Accessed: 15th January 2016].

Framingham Heart Study. (n.d.) (2) Research Milestones. [Online] Available from: https://www.framinghamheartstudy.org/about-fhs/research-milestones. php [Accessed: 15th January 2016].

Gardner, C. D. et al. (2007) Comparison of the Atkins, Zone, Ornish, and LEARN Diets for Change in Weight and Related Risk Factors Among Overweight Premenopausal Women. The Journal of the American Medical Association [Online] Vol 297, No. 9. Available from: http://jama.jamanetwork.com/article.aspx?articleid=205916 [Accessed: 15th January 2016].

Geoba.se (2015). The World: Life Expectancy (2015) – Top 100+. [Online] Available from: http://www.geoba.se/population.php?pc=world&page=1&type=15&st=rank&asde=&year=2015 [Accessed: 15th January 2016].

Georgia State University News. (2015) Widely Used Food Additive Promotes Colitis, Obesity and Metabolic Syndrome. [Online] 26th February. Available from: http://news.gsu.edu/2015/02/26/widely-used-food-additive-promotes-colitis-obesity-metabolic-syndrome-research-shows/ [Accessed: 15th January 2016].

Gilbert, N. (2012) Rapeseed biodiesel fails sustainability test. Nature. [Online] 9th August. Available from: http://www.nature.com/news/rapeseed-biodiesel-fails-sustainability-test-1.11145 [Accessed: 15th January 2016].

Giordani, M. (2014) Total Joint Arthroplasty. [Online] Available from: http://www.ucdmc.ucdavis.edu/minimed/pdfs/2014_02_08_Total_Joint_Arthroplasty_M_GiordaniMD.pdf [Accessed: 15th January 2016].

Gladwell, M. (2008) Outliers: The Story of Success. New York: Little, Brown and Company.

Goff, J. (2012) Q&A with Dr. Goff. Fatty Liver Disease. [Online] Available from: http://www.liverfoundation.org/chapters/rockymountain/doctorsnotes/article1/ [Accessed: 15th January 2016].

Goldacre, B. (2007) Science and Fiction. New Statesman. [Online] 27th January, p.16. Available from: http://www.badscience.net/2007/01/science-and-fiction/ [Accessed: 15th January 2016].

Goleman, D. (1995) Emotional Intelligence: Why It Can Matter More Than IQ. London: Bantam Books.

Gunnars, K. (2013) 6 Reasons why vegetable oils can be harmful. Authority Nutrition. [Online] August 2013. Available from: http://authoritynutrition.com/6-reasons-why-vegetable-oils-are-toxic/ [Accessed: 15th January 2016].

Harcombe, Z. et al. (2015) Evidence from randomised controlled trials did not support the introduction of dietary fat guidelines in 1977 and 1983: a systematic review and meta-analysis. Open Heart. [Online] 2015 Jan 29;2(1):e000196.

Available from: http://www.ncbi.nlm.nih.gov/pubmed/25685363 [Accessed: 15th January 2016].

Harris, D. R. (ed.) (1996) The origins and spread of pastoralism in Eurasia. London: UCL Press.

Harvard Health Publications, Harvard Medical School. (2011) When the liver gets fatty. [Online] Available from: http://www.health.harvard.edu/diseases-and-conditions/when-the-liver-gets-fatty [Accessed: 15th January 2016].

Harvard T.H. Chan School of Public Health. (2015) Waking Up to Sleep's Role in Weight Control. [Online] Available from: http://www.hsph.harvard.edu/obesity-prevention-source/obesity-causes/sleep-and-obesity/ [Accessed: 15th January 2016].

Hawks, J. (2013) How Has the Human Brain Evolved? [Online] 1st July. Available from: http://www.scientificamerican.com/article/how-has-human-brain-evolved/ [Accessed: 15th January 2016].

Heath, D. and Heath, C. (2007) Made to Stick. New York: Random House.

Heid, M. (2015) Why Full-Fat Dairy May Be Healthier Than Low-Fat. Time Magazine. [Online] 5th March. Available from: http://time.com/3734033/whole-milk-dairy-fat/ [Accessed: 15th January 2016].

Heymsfield, S. B. et al. (1999) Recombinant Leptin for Weight Loss in Obese and Lean Adults. Journal of the American Medical Association. [Online] Vol 282, No. 16. Available from: http://jama.jamanetwork.com/article.aspx?articleid=192037&resultclick=1 [Accessed: 15th January 2016].

Hoenselaar, R. (2011) Consumption of dietary saturated fat and cardiovascular disease. [Online] Available from: http://canceranddiet.nl/cardiovascular_disease/saturated-fat.html [Accessed: 15th January 2016].

Holmberg, S. et al. (2009) Food Choices and Coronary Heart Disease. Int. J. Environ. Res. Public Health [Online] 2009,6(10), 2626-2638. Available from: http://www.mdpi.com/1660-4601/6/10/2626/htm [Accessed: 15th January 2016].

Hunt-Peters, L. (1918) Diet and Health: With Key to the Calories. Chicago: The Reilly and Lee Co.

Husten, L. (2015) CardioBrief: Second Opinion on BMJ Dietary Guideline Takedown - What do other experts say on critique of the proposed U.S. dietary guidelines? Medpage Today. [Online] 25th September. Available from: http://www.medpagetoday.com/Cardiology/CardioBrief/53723 [Accessed: 15th January 2016].

IANS. (2015) 9 of world's 10 most obese countries are in the Pacific. The Times of India. [Online] 12th May 2015. Available from: http://timesofindia.indiatimes.com/life-style/health-fitness/weight-loss/9-of-worlds-10-most-obese-countries-are-in-the-Pacific/articleshow/47247649.cms [Accessed: 15th January 2016].

Imhoff, D. (2010) The CAFO Reader: The Tragedy of Industrial Animal Feeding Factories. Berkeley, California: University of California Press.

International Diabetes Federation. (2013) Western Pacific Action Plan Launched. [Online] Available from: http://www.idf.org/western-pacific-action-plan-launched [Accessed: 15th January 2016].

Jönsson, T. et al. (2009) Beneficial effects of a Paleolithic diet on cardiovascular risk factors in type 2 diabetes: a randomized cross-over pilot study. Cardiovasc Diabetol. [Online] 2009; 8: 35. Available from: http://www.ncbi.nlm.nih.gov/pmc/articles/PMC2724493/ [Accessed: 15th January 2016].

Jou, C. (2015) Counting Calories. Chemical Heritage Magazine. [Online] Available from: http://www.chemheritage.org/discover/media/magazine/articles/29-1-counting-calories.aspx [Accessed: 15th January 2016].

Kahnemann, D. (2011) Thinking, Fast and Slow. New York: Farrar, Straus and Giroux.

Keene, D. et al. (2014) Effect on cardiovascular risk of high density lipoprotein targeted drug treatments niacin, fibrates, and CETP inhibitors: meta-analysis of randomised controlled trials including 117 411 patients. BMJ [Online] 2014;349:g4379. Available from: http://www.bmj.com/content/349/bmj.g4379 [Accessed: 15th January 2016].

Ketogenic Diet Resource. (n.d.) Low Carb Diet Side Effects. [Online] Available from: http://www.ketogenic-diet-resource.com/low-carb-diet-side-effects.html [Accessed: 15th January 2016].

Keys, A. (1950) The Biology of Human Starvation. Minneapolis, University of Minnesota Press.

Keys, A. (1966) Arteriosclerotic heart disease in a favored community. Journal of Clinical Epidemiology. [Online] Volume 19, Issue 3, Pages 245–254. Available from: http://www.jclinepi.com/article/0021-9681(66)90130-5/abstract [Accessed: 15th January 2016].

Keys, A. et al. (1972) Indices of relative weight and obesity. Journal of Chronic Diseases. [Online] Vol 25 Issues 6-7, July 1972, pp329–343. Available from: http://www.sciencedirect.com/science/article/pii/0021968172900276 [Accessed: 15th January 2016].

Knopp, R. and Retzlaff, B. (2004) Saturated fat prevents coronary artery disease? An American paradox. Am J Clin Nutr [Online] November 2004 vol. 80 no. 5 1102-1103. Available from: http://ajcn.nutrition.org/content/80/5/1102.full [Accessed: 15th January 2016].

Kovacs, J. S. (2009) The Dos and Don'ts of Counting Calories. WebMD. [Online] 4th February 2009. Available from: http://www.webmd.com/diet/dos-donts-counting-calories [Accessed: 15th January 2016].

Kratz, M. et al. (2013) The relationship between high-fat dairy consumption and obesity, cardiovascular, and metabolic disease. Eur J Nutr. [Online] 2013 Feb;52(1):1–24. Available from: http://www.ncbi.nlm.nih.gov/pubmed/22810464 [Accessed: 15th January 2016].

Kummerow, F.A. (2013) Correlation between oxysterol consumption and heart disease. Clinical Lipidology. [Online] Vol. 8, No. 3, Pages 289-294. Available from: http://www.futuremedicine.com/doi/full/10.2217/clp.13.34 [Accessed: 15th January 2016].

Lancaster, H. O. (1990) Expectations of Life: A Study in the Demography, Statistics, and History of World Mortality. New York: Springer Verlag.

Lawrence, F. (2008) Eat Your Heart Out. London: Penguin.

Lee, S. (2009) Glucose Shortens the Lifespan of Caenorhabditis elegans by Down-Regulating Aquaporin Gene Expression. Cell Metab. [Online] 2009 Nov; 10(5): 379–391. Available from: http://www.ncbi.nlm.nih.gov/pmc/articles/PMC2887095/ [Accessed: 15th January 2016].

Levy, B. R. (2002) Longevity increased by positive self-perceptions of aging. J Pers Soc Psychol. [Online] 2002 Aug;83(2):261-70. Available from: http://www.ncbi.nlm.nih.gov/pubmed/12150226 [Accessed: 15th January 2016].

Light, L. (2004) A Fatally Flawed Food Guide. [Online] Available from: http://www.whale.to/a/light.html [Accessed: 15th January 2016].

Lindeberg, S. et al. (2007) A Paleolithic diet improves glucose tolerance more than a Mediterranean-like diet in individuals with ischaemic heart disease. Diabetologia. [Online] September 2007, Volume 50, Issue 9, pp. 1795–1807. Available from: http://www.springerlink.com/content/h7628r66r0552222 [Accessed: 15th January 2016].

Loyola University Health System. (2015) Exercise alone does not help in losing weight. Science Daily. [Online] 7th August. Available from: www.sciencedaily.com/releases/2015/08/150817142140.htm [Accessed: 15th January 2016].

Lund University (2015) High-fat dairy products linked to reduced type 2 diabetes risk. Science Daily. [Online] 2nd April. Available from: http://www.sciencedaily.com/releases/2015/04/150402081804.htm [Accessed: 15th January 2016].

Lustig, R. (2013) Fructose: the poison index. The Guardian. [Online] 21st October. Available from: http://www.theguardian.com/commentisfree/2013/oct/21/fructose-poison-sugar-industry-pseudoscience [Accessed: 15th January 2016].

Mabuchi, H. et al. (2002) Large scale cohort study of the relationship between serum cholesterol concentration and coronary events with low-dose simvastatin therapy in Japanese patients with hypercholesterolemia and coronary heart disease: secondary prevention cohort study of the Japan Lipid Intervention Trial (J-LIT). Circ J. [Online] 2002 Dec;66(12):1096–100. Available from: http://www.ncbi.nlm.nih.gov/pubmed/12499612 [Accessed: 15th January 2016].

Mackarness, R. (1959) Eat Fat and Grow Slim. Garden City, New York: Doubleday.

Malhotra, A. (2013) Saturated fat is not the major issue. BMJ [Online] 2013;347:f6340. Available from: http://www.bmj.com/content/347/bmj.f6340 [Accessed: 15th January 2016].

Mattson, Mark P. (2005). Energy Intake, Meal Frequency, and Health: A Neurobiological Perspective. Annu Rev Nutr. [Online] 2005;25:237–60. Available from: http://www.ncbi.nlm.nih.gov/pubmed/16011467 [Accessed: 15th January 2016].

Mayo. (2013) S. Stanley Young: Scientific Integrity and Transparency. [Online] 11th March 2013. Available from: http://errorstatistics.com/2013/03/11/s-stanley-young-scientific-integrity-and-transparency/ [Accessed: 15th January 2016].

McCarrison, R. (1921) Studies in Deficiency Disease. London: Hodder & Stoughton.

McClellan, W.S. and Du Bois, E.F. (1930) Prolonged meat diets with a study of kidney function and ketosis. Journal of Biological Chemistry. [Online] July 1, 1930, 87, 651-668. Available from: http://www.jbc.org/content/87/3/651.full.pdf+html [Accessed: 15th January 2016].

Messinger, L. (2015) Could low-fat be worse for you than whole milk? The Guardian. [Online] 9th October. Available from: http://www.theguardian.com/lifeandstyle/2015/oct/09/low-fat-whole-milk-usda-dietary-guidelines [Accessed: 15th January 2016].

Metz, E. (2015) Does Cadbury chocolate taste different in different countries? BBC News Magazine. [Online] 18th March. Available from: http://www.bbc.com/news/magazine-31924912 [Accessed: 15th January 2016].

Miller, D. W. (2015) Fallacies in Modern Medicine: Statins and the Cholesterol-Heart Hypothesis. Journal of American Physicians and Surgeons. [Online] Vol 20, No 2. Available from: http://www.jpands.org/vol20no2/miller.pdf [Accessed: 15th January 2016].

Minger, D. (2014) Death by Food Pyramid: How Shoddy Science, Sketchy Politics and Shady Special Interests Have Ruined Our Health. Malibu, CA: Primal Blueprint Publishing.

Morell, S.F. (2005) Dirty Secrets of the Food Processing Industry. [Online] 26th December 2005. Available from: http://www.westonaprice.org/health-topics/dirty-secrets-of-the-food-processing-industry/ [Accessed: 15th January 2016].

Morrell, S. F. and Daniel, K. T. (2014) Nourishing Broth. New York: Grand Central Life & Style.

Moss, G.E. (2011) The Dawning Age of Cooperation: The End of Civilization as We Know It … and Just in Time. New York: Algora Publishing.

Mozaffarian, D. et al., (2011) Changes in Diet and Lifestyle and Long-Term Weight Gain in Women and Men. N Engl J Med [Online] 2011; 364:2392-2404. Available from: http://www.nejm.org/doi/full/10.1056/NEJMoa1014296 [Accessed: 15th January 2016].

Muraki, I. et al. (2013) Fruit consumption and risk of type 2 diabetes: results from three prospective longitudinal cohort studies. BMJ [Online] 2013;347:f5001. Available from: http://www.bmj.com/content/347/bmj.f5001 [Accessed: 15th January 2016].

Nago, N. et al. (2011) Low cholesterol is associated with mortality from stroke, heart disease, and cancer: the Jichi Medical School Cohort Study. J Epidemiol. [Online] 2011;21(1):67–74. Available from: http://www.ncbi.nlm.nih.gov/pubmed/21160131 [Accessed: 15th January 2016].

National Heart, Lung, and Blood Institute. (2005) Honolulu Heart Program (HHP). [Online] Available from: https://biolincc.nhlbi.nih.gov/studies/hhp/ [Accessed: 15th January 2016].

National Resources Defense Council. (n.d.) Food, Farm Animals and Drugs. [Online] Available from: http://www.nrdc.org/food/saving-antibiotics.asp [Accessed: 15th January 2016].

Nestle, M. (2015) Never a dull moment: the BMJ's attack on the Dietary Guidelines Advisory Committee report. Food Politics. [Online] 28th September. Available from: http://www.foodpolitics.com/2015/09/never-a-dull-moment-the-bmjs-attack-on-the-dietary-guidelines-advisory-committee-report/ [Accessed: 15th January 2016].

Nestle, M. and Nesheim, M. (2013) Why Calories Count: From Science to Politics. Berkeley, California: University of California Press.

Ng, S. W. et al. (2012) Use of caloric and noncaloric sweeteners in US consumer packaged foods, 2005-2009. J Acad Nutr Diet. [Online] 2012 Nov;112(11). Available from: http://www.ncbi.nlm.nih.gov/pubmed/23102182 [Accessed: 15th January 2016].

NHS (2014) Eat a balanced diet. [Online] Available from: http://www.nhs.uk/Livewell/Goodfood/Pages/Healthyeating.aspx [Accessed: 15th January 2016].

NHS (2015) (1) 5 A DAY. [Online] Available from: http://www.nhs.uk/livewell/5aday/Pages/5ADAYhome.aspx [Accessed: 15th January 2016].

NHS (2015) (2) High cholesterol. [Online] Available from: http://www.nhs.uk/conditions/Cholesterol/Pages/Introduction.aspx [Accessed: 15th January 2016].

Novotny, J. A. et al. (2012) Discrepancy between the Atwater factor predicted and empirically measured energy values of almonds in human diets. Am J Clin Nutr. [Online] 3rd July 2012. Available from: http://ajcn.nutrition.org/content/early/2012/06/28/ajcn.112.035782.full.pdf+html [Accessed: 15th January 2016].

Nowbar A. N. et al. (2014) Global geographic analysis of mortality from ischaemic heart disease. International Journal of Cardiology. [Online] June 15, 2014. Volume 174, Issue 2, Pages 293–298. Available from: http://www.internationaljournalofcardiology.com/article/S0167-5273(14)00755-4/fulltext [Accessed: 15th January 2016].

NuSI. (n.d.) Pediatric Nonalcoholic Fatty Liver Disease Study. [Online] Available from: http://nusi.org/science-in-progress/nonalcoholic-fatty-liver-disease-study/ [Accessed: 15th January 2016].

O'Connor, A. (2015) Nutrition Panel Calls for Less Sugar and Eases Cholesterol and Fat Restrictions. [Online] 19th February 2015. Available from: http://well.blogs.nytimes.com/2015/02/19/nutrition-panel-calls-for-less-sugar-and-eases-cholesterol-and-fat-restrictions/ [Accessed: 15th January 2016].

O'Connor, A. (2015) What Eating 40 Teaspoons of Sugar a Day Can Do to You. [Online] 14th August 2015. Available from: http://well.blogs.nytimes.com/2015/08/14/what-eating-40-teaspoons-of-sugar-a-day-can-do-to-you/ [Accessed: 15th January 2016].

OECD. (2007) Agricultural Policies in OECD Countries 2007. [Online] Available from: http://www.oecd.org/tad/agricultural-policies/39524780.pdf [Accessed: 15th January 2016].

Ogden, C. L. et al. (2004) Mean Body Weight, Height, And Body Mass Index. Advance Data from Vital and Health Statistics. [Online] Number 347, October 27, 2004. Available from: http://www.cdc.gov/nchs/data/ad/ad347.pdf [Accessed: 15th January 2016].

O'Keefe, S. J. D. et al. (2014) Fat, Fibre and cancer risk in African Americans and rural Africans. Nature Communications. [Online] 6, 6342. 28 April 2015. Available from: http://www.nature.com/ncomms/2015/150428/ncomms7342/full/ncomms7342.html [Accessed: 15th January 2016].

Oregon State University. (2015) Fat, sugar cause bacterial changes that may relate to loss of cognitive function. [Online] 22nd June 2015. Available from: http://oregonstate.edu/ua/ncs/archives/2015/jun/fat-sugar-cause-bacterial-changes-may-relate-loss-cognitive-function [Accessed: 15th January 2016].

O'Riordan, M. (2014) No Clinical Benefit to Raising HDL With Existing Therapies, Meta-Analysis Shows. Medscape. [Online] 23rd July 2014. Available from: http://www.medscape.com/viewarticle/828779 [Accessed: 15th January 2016].

Otto, M. et al. (2012) Dietary intake of saturated fat by food source and incident cardiovascular disease: the Multi-Ethnic Study of Atherosclerosis. AJCN. [Online] 3rd July. Available from: http://ajcn.nutrition.org/content/early/2012/06/28/ajcn.112.037770.full.pdf+html [Accessed: 15th January 2016].

Otto, M. et al. (2013) Biomarkers of Dairy Fatty Acids and Risk of Cardiovascular Disease in the Multi-Ethnic Study of Atherosclerosis. J Am Heart Assoc. [Online] 18th July. Available from: http://jaha.ahajournals.org/content/2/4/e000092.full [Accessed: 15th January 2016].

Paddock, C. (2014) Prolonged fasting 're-boots' immune system. Medical News Today. [Online] 6th June. Available from: http://www.medicalnewstoday.com/articles/277860.php [Accessed: 15th January 2016].

Parretti, H. et al. (2015) Efficacy of water preloading before main meals as a strategy for weight loss in primary care patients with obesity: RCT. Obesity. [Online] Volume 23, Issue 9. pp. 1785–1791. Available from: http://onlinelibrary.wiley.com/doi/10.1002/oby.21167/abstract [Accessed: 15th January 2016].

Paturel, A. (2015) The Ultimate Arthritis Diet. [Online] Available from: http://www.arthritis.org/living-with-arthritis/arthritis-diet/anti-inflammatory/the-arthritis-diet.php [Accessed: 15th January 2016].

Petroni, S. (2015) Daily Sugar Drinks Can Lead to Liver Disease. Patch. [Online] 12th June. Available from: http://patch.com/massachusetts/framingham/study-daily-sugar-drinks-can-lead-liver-disease-0 [Accessed: 15th January 2016].

Pollan, M. (2006) Six Rules For Eating Wisely. TIME Magazine. [Online] 4th June. Available from: http://michaelpollan.com/articles-archive/six-rules-for-eating-wisely/ [Accessed: 15th January 2016].

Pollan, M. (2007) Unhappy Meals. The New York Times Magazine, [Online] 28th January. Available from: http://michaelpollan.com/articles-archive/un-happy-meals/ [Accessed: 15th January 2016].

Pollan, M. (2008) In Defense of Food. New York: Penguin Press.

Positano, R. (2008) The Mystery of the Rosetan People. Huffington Post. [Online] 28th March 2008. Available from: http://www.huffingtonpost.com/dr-rock-positano/the-mystery-of-the-roseta_b_73260.html [Accessed: 15th January 2016].

Rasmussen, W. D. and Stone, P. S. (1982) Toward a Third Agricultural Revolution. Proceedings of the Academy of Political Science. v34 n3 (19820101):174–185.

Rettner, R. (2013) Calorie Labels Inaccurate, Experts Say. [Online] 1st February. Available from: http://www.livescience.com/26799-calorie-counts-inaccurate.html [Accessed: 15th January 2016].

Richards, F. (1939) Billy Bunter's Bargain Magnet #1659. [Online] Available from: http://www.friardale.co.uk/Magnet/1939/Magnet%201659-A.pdf [Accessed: 15th January 2016].

Rimm, E.B. et al. (1996) Vegetable, fruit, and cereal fiber intake and risk of coronary heart disease among men. JAMA. [Online] 1996 Feb 14;275(6):447–51. Available from: http://www.ncbi.nlm.nih.gov/pubmed/8627965 [Accessed: 15th January 2016].

Robert Wood Johnson Foundation. (2015) Adult Obesity in the United States. [Online] Available from: http://stateofobesity.org/adult-obesity/ [Accessed: 15th January 2016].

Rossen, J. and Powell, R. (2012) Rossen Reports: Can you believe diet frozen dessert labels? Today. [Online] 20th August 2012. Available from: http://www.today.com/id/48596412/ns/today-today_news/t/rossen-reports-can-you-believe-diet-frozen-dessert-labels/#.Vm1tOPkrKhc [Accessed: 15th January 2016].

Russ, T. C. et al. (2012) Association between psychological distress and mortality: individual participant pooled analysis of 10 prospective cohort studies. BMJ [Online] 2012;345:e4933. Available from: http://www.bmj.com/content/345/bmj.e4933 [Accessed: 15th January 2016].

Schatz, I. J. et al. (2001) Cholesterol and all-cause mortality in elderly people from the Honolulu Heart Program: a cohort study. Lancet. [Online] 2001

Aug 4;358(9279):351-5. Available from: http://www.ncbi.nlm.nih.gov/pubmed/11502313 [Accessed: 15th January 2016].

Schofield, G. (2015) 5 reasons sugar, not fat is the problem. [Online] Available from: http://profgrant.com/2015/07/21/5-reasons-sugar-not-fat-is-the-problem/ [Accessed: 15th January 2016].

Shanahan, C. (2009) Deep Nutrition. Lawai, HI: Big Books.

Sheth, S. G. and Chopra, S. (2015) Epidemiology, clinical features, and diagnosis of nonalcoholic fatty liver disease in adults. [Online] Available from: http://www.uptodate.com/contents/epidemiology-clinical-features-and-diagnosis-of-nonalcoholic-fatty-liver-disease-in-adults [Accessed: 15th January 2016].

Sigurdsson, A. F. (2015) Cholesterol and Heart Disease – A Quick Look Beyond. [Online] 18th January 2015. Available from: http://www.docsopinion.com/2015/01/18/cholesterol-and-heart-disease-a-quick-look-beyond/ [Accessed: 15th January 2016].

Simopoulos, A. P. (2002) The importance of the ratio of omega-6/omega-3 essential fatty acids. Biomed Pharmacother. [Online] 2002 Oct;56(8):365-79. Available from: http://www.ncbi.nlm.nih.gov/pubmed/12442909 [Accessed: 15th January 2016].

Siri-Tarino, P.W. et al. (2010). Meta-analysis of prospective cohort studies evaluating the association of saturated fat with cardiovascular disease. Am J Clin Nutr [Online] 13th January 2010, ajcn.27725. Available from: http://ajcn.nutrition.org/content/early/2010/01/13/ajcn.2009.27725.full.pdf+html [Accessed: 15th January 2016].

Smith, M. (2007) Here's to a healthier heart. The Guardian. [Online] 30th October 2007. Available from: http://www.theguardian.com/lifeandstyle/2007/oct/30/healthandwellbeing.health [Accessed: 15th January 2016].

Sofi, F. et al. (2014) Effect of Triticum turgidum subsp. turanicum wheat on irritable bowel syndrome: a double-blinded randomised dietary intervention trial. Br J Nutr. [Online] 2014 Feb 13:1-8. Available from: http://www.ncbi.nlm.nih.gov/pubmed/24521561 [Accessed: 15th January 2016].

Spalding, K. et al. (2008) Dynamics of fat cell turnover in humans. Nature [Online] 453, 783-787 (5 June 2008). Available from: http://www.nature.com/nature/journal/v453/n7196/abs/nature06902.html [Accessed: 15th January 2016].

Spector, T. (2012) Identically Different: Why You Can Change Your Genes. London: Weidenfield & Nicolson.

Spector, T. (2015) The Diet Myth: The Real Science Behind What We Eat. London: Weidenfield & Nicolson.

Stampone, J. (2011) The Roseto Effect – The Valley of the Roses. [Online] 24th June 2011. Available from: http://yocuzlawyers.com/2011/06/the-roseto-effect-the-valley-of-the-roses [Accessed: 15th January 2016].

Stanford Hospital and Clinics. (2015) The Low FODMAP Diet (FODMAP=-Fermentable Oligo-Di-Monosaccharides and Polyols). [Online] Available from: https://stanfordhealthcare.org/content/dam/SHC/for-patients-component/programs-services/clinical-nutrition-services/docs/pdf-lowfodmapdiet.pdf [Accessed: 15th January 2016].

Stare, F. J. (1973) Summary of symposium and recommendations for food industry action. Preventive Medicine, [Online] Volume 2, Issue 3, Pages 407-411. Available from: http://www.sciencedirect.com/science/article/pii/0091743573900376 [Accessed: 15th January 2016].

Stare, F. J. et al. (1989) Balanced Nutrition: Beyond the Cholestrol Scare. Holbrook, MA: B. Adams.

Stephens, A. (2009) The vegetables that can hydrate you more than a glass of water. The Daily Mail. [Online] 18th July. Available from: http://www.dailymail.co.uk/health/article-1200531/The-vegetables-hydrate-glass-water.html [Accessed: 15th January 2016].

Stitt, P. A. (1982) Beating the Food Giants. Manitowoc, WI: Natural Press.

Stoye, E. (2015) Simple cooking changes make healthier rice. Chemistry World. [Online] 23rd March. Available from: http://www.rsc.org/chemistry-world/2015/03/low-calorie-healthy-rice-resistant-starch [Accessed: 15th January 2016].

Stulp, G. et al. (2015) Does natural selection favour taller stature among the tallest people on earth? The Royal Society Publishing Proceedings B. [Online] Available from: http://rspb.royalsocietypublishing.org/content/282/1806/20150211 [Accessed: 15th January 2016].

Sumner, D. A. (2008) Agricultural subsidy programs. In Henderson, D. R. (ed.) The Concise Encyclopedia of Economics. Liberty Fund, Inc. Library of Economics and Liberty. [Online] Available from: http://www.econlib.org/library/Enc/AgriculturalSubsidyPrograms.html [Accessed: 15th January 2016].

Super Size Me (2004) Film. Directed by Morgan Spurlock. [DVD] New York: Hart Sharp Video.

Szwarc, S. (2008) I think, therefore I am: Part One. [Online] 16th February 2008. Available from: http://junkfoodscience.blogspot.be/2008/02/i-think-therefore-i-am-part-one.html [Accessed: 15th January 2016].

Taranu, I. et al. (2014) Omega-3 PUFA Rich Camelina Oil By-Products Improve the Systemic Metabolism and Spleen Cell Functions in Fattening Pigs. PLoS One. [Online] 2014; 9(10): e110186. Available from: http://www.ncbi. nlm.nih.gov/pmc/articles/PMC4193896/ [Accessed: 15th January 2016].

Taubes, G. (2008) Good Calories, Bad Calories: Fats, Carbs, and the Controversial Science of Diet and Health. New York: Anchor Books.

Taylor, R. (2015) Further information on the research on Reversing Type 2 Diabetes. [Online] Available from: http://www.ncl.ac.uk/magres/research/diabetes/documents/Diabetes-Reversaloftype2study%20June%2015.pdf [Accessed: 15th January 2016].

TEDMED. (2013) Peter Attia: Is the obesity crisis hiding a bigger problem? [Online video]. April 2013. Available from: https://www.ted.com/talks/peter_attia_what_if_we_re_wrong_about_diabetes [Accessed: 15th January 2016].

Teicholz, N. (2014) The Big Fat Surprise: Why Butter, Meat and Cheese Belong in a Healthy Diet. New York: Simon & Schuster.

Teicholz, N. (2015) (1) The Government's Bad Diet Advice. The New York Times. [Online] 20th February. Available from: http://www.nytimes. com/2015/02/21/opinion/when-the-government-tells-you-what-to-eat.html [Accessed: 15th January 2016].

Teicholz, N. (2015) (2) The scientific report guiding the US dietary guidelines: is it scientific? BMJ [Online] 2015;351:h4962. Available from: http://www. bmj.com/content/351/bmj.h4962 [Accessed: 15th January 2016].

Telis, G. (2013) Lard may not be as bad for your health as the fat's detractors say. The Washington Post. [Online] 15th April. Available from: https:// www.washingtonpost.com/national/health-science/lard-may-not-be-as-bad-for-your-health-as-the-fats-detractors-say/2013/04/15/874490a0-9bb5-11e2-9bda-edd1a7fb557d_story.html [Accessed: 15th January 2016].

Tenderich, A. (2012) Carbs or Fat: What Really Makes Us Gain Weight? (Guest Post by Jessica Apple). [Online] Available from: http://www.healthline. com/diabetesmine/carbs-or-fat-what-really-makes-us-gain-weight#1 [Accessed: 15th January 2016].

That Sugar Film. (2014) Film. Directed by Damon Gameau. [DVD] Victoria: Madman Entertainment Pty Ltd.

The Cutting Factory. (2015) Sugar Coated [Online video] 23rd October. Available from: https://vimeo.com/ondemand/sugarcoated/143152323 [Accessed: 15th January 2016].

The Dairy Council. (n.d.) The principles of a healthy balanced diet explained. [Online] Available from: http://www.milk.co.uk/page.aspx?intPageID=129 [Accessed: 15th January 2016].

The Guardian. (2015) Most liver transplants by 2020 will be 'linked to over-eating, not alcohol'. The Guardian. [Online] 3rd May. Available from: http://www.theguardian.com/society/2015/may/03/most-liver-transplants-linked-to-over-eating-not-alcohol [Accessed: 15th January 2016].

TheSceneLab. (2014) Carb-Loaded: A Culture Dying to Eat. [Online Video]. 28th August 2015. Available from: https://vimeo.com/ondemand/carbloaded [Accessed: 15th January 2016].

Trust Me, I'm A Doctor. Series 3, Episode 3: Could your cooking oils be damaging your health? (2015) BBC Two, 29th July 2015.

UNdata. (2012 revision) Infant Mortality Rate. [Online] Available from: http://data.un.org/Data.aspx?d=PopDiv&f=variableID%3A77#PopDiv [Accessed: 15th January 2016].

United States Department of Agriculture. (2015) Scientific Report of the 2015 Dietary Guidelines Advisory Committee. [Online] Available from: http://health.gov/dietaryguidelines/2015-scientific-report/pdfs/scientific-report-of-the-2015-dietary-guidelines-advisory-committee.pdf [Accessed: 15th January 2016].

University of Manchester. (2010) Scientists suggest that cancer is man-made. [Online] Available from: http://www.manchester.ac.uk/discover/news/scientists-suggest-that-cancer-is-man-made [Accessed: 15th January 2016].

Unwin, D. and Tobin, S. (2015) A patient request for some "deprescribing". BMJ [Online] 2015;351:h4023. Available from: http://www.bmj.com/content/351/bmj.h4023 [Accessed: 15th January 2016].

US Food and Drug Administration. (2015) FDA Cuts Trans Fat in Processed Foods. [Online] Available from: http://www.fda.gov/ForConsumers/ConsumerUpdates/ucm372915.htm [Accessed: 15th January 2016].

USDA Economic Research Service. (2015) Food Availability and Consumption. [Online] Available from: http://www.ers.usda.gov/data-products/ag-and-food-statistics-charting-the-essentials/food-availability-and-consumption.aspx [Accessed: 15th January 2016].

USDA National Agricultural Library. (n.d.) MyPlate and Historical Food Pyramid Resources. [Online] Available from: http://fnic.nal.usda.gov/dietary-guidance/myplate-and-historical-food-pyramid-resources [Accessed: 15th January 2016].

Valtin, H. (2002) "Drink at least eight glasses of water a day." Really? Is there scientific evidence for "8 × 8"? American Journal of Physiology - Regulatory, Integrative and Comparative Physiology. [Online] Nov 2002, 283 (5) R993-R1004. Available from: http://ajpregu.physiology.org/content/283/5/R993 [Accessed: 15th January 2016].

Ventura, E.E. et al. (2010) Sugar Content of Popular Sweetened Beverages Based on Objective Laboratory Analysis: Focus on Fructose Content. Obesity [Online] (October 2010). Available from: http://goranlab.com/pdf/Ventura%20Obesity%202010-sugary%20beverages.pdf [Accessed: 15th January 2016].

Viadecouvertesprod. (2011) The Science of Fasting. [Online video]. 14th November 2011. Available from: https://www.youtube.com/watch?v=sNdWC-ZWpjxU [Accessed: 15th January 2016].

Virginia Tech. (2015) Scientists reveal cellular clockwork underlying inflammation. Science Daily. [Online] 27th August 2015. Available from: http://www.sciencedaily.com/releases/2015/08/150827130137.htm [Accessed: 15th January 2016].

Volek et al. (2011) The Art and Science of Low Carbohydrate Living. Lexington, KY: Beyond Obesity.

WebMD (2014) Fatty Liver Disease. [Online] Available from: http://www.webmd.com/hepatitis/fatty-liver-disease [Accessed: 15th January 2016].

Wheless, J. W. (2004) History and Origin of the Ketogenic Diet. In Stafstrom, C. E. and Rho, J. M. (eds.) Epilepsy and the Ketogenic Diet. Totowa, NJ: Humana Press Inc. [Online] Available from: http://www.naturaleater.com/science-articles/history-ketogenic-diet.pdf [Accessed: 15th January 2016].

Which? Magazine. (2015) Revealed: the salads and sandwiches with more fat than a burger. Which? News. [Online] 17th April. Available from: http://www.which.co.uk/news/2015/04/revealed-the-salads-and-sandwiches-with-more-fat-than-a-burger-400480/ [Accessed: 15th January 2016].

Whoriskey, P. (2015) (1). The science of skipping breakfast: How government nutritionists may have gotten it wrong. [Online] 10th August 2015. Available from: https://www.washingtonpost.com/news/wonk/wp/2015/08/10/the-science-of-skipping-breakfast-how-government-nutritionists-may-have-gotten-it-wrong/ [Accessed: 15th January 2016].

Whoriskey, P. (2015) (2) For decades, the government steered millions away from whole milk. Was that wrong? [Online] 6th October 2015. Available from: https://www.washingtonpost.com/news/wonk/wp/2015/10/06/for-decades-the-government-steered-millions-away-from-whole-milk-was-that-wrong/ [Accessed: 15th January 2016].

Wikipedia. (n.d.) (1) Robert Atkins (nutritionist). [Online] Available from: https://en.wikipedia.org/wiki/Robert_Atkins_(nutritionist) [Accessed: 15th January 2016].

Wikipedia. n.d. (2) Granula. [Online] Available from: https://en.wikipedia.org/wiki/Granula [Accessed: 15th January 2016].

Willett, W. et al. (1987) Dietary Fat and the Risk of Breast Cancer. N Engl J Med [Online] 1987; 316:22-28. Available from: http://www.nejm.org/doi/full/10.1056/NEJM198701013160105 [Accessed: 15th January 2016].

Williams, P.T. and Wood, P. D. (2006) The effects of changing exercise levels on weight and age-related weight gain. Int J Obes (Lond). [Online] 2006 Mar; 30(3): 543–551. Available from: http://www.ncbi.nlm.nih.gov/pmc/articles/PMC2864590/ [Accessed: 15th January 2016].

Winterman, D. (2012) Breakfast, lunch and dinner: Have we always eaten them? BBC News Magazine. [Online] 15th November 2012. Available from: http://www.bbc.com/news/magazine-20243692 [Accessed: 15th January 2016].

Wolf, S. and Bruhn, J. G. (1993) The Power of Clan: The Influence of Human Relationships on Heart Disease. New Brunswick, N.J.: Transaction Publishers.

Wolf, S. et al. (1989) Roseto, Pennsylvania 25 years later--highlights of a medical and sociological survey. Trans Am Clin Climatol Assoc. [Online] 1989; 100: 57–67. Available from: http://www.ncbi.nlm.nih.gov/pmc/articles/PMC2376462/ [Accessed: 15th January 2016].

World Health Organization. (1948) Preamble to the Constitution of the World Health Organization as adopted by the International Health Conference, New York, 19-22 June, 1946. [Online] Available from: http://www.who.int/about/definition/en/print.html [Accessed: 15th January 2016].

Wrangham, R. (2009) Catching Fire: How Cooking Made Us Human. London: Profile Books.

Yellowlees, W. (1983) Modern diseases, seen from a Highland practice. An ecological approach. Ecology of Disease. [Online] 02/1983; 2(1):81-91. Available from: https://www.researchgate.net/publication/16864295_Modern_diseases_seen_from_a_Highland_practice_An_ecological_approach [Accessed: 15th January 2016].

Yerushalmy, J. and Hilleboe, H. (1957) Fat in the diet and mortality from heart disease; a methodologic note. New York State Journal of Medicine. [Online] Extracts available from: http://www.epi.umn.edu/cvdepi/essay/famous-polemics-on-diet-heart-theory/ [Accessed: 15th January 2016].

Yudkin, J. (1972) Pure, White and Deadly. London: Davis-Poynter Ltd.

LIST OF WEBSITES REFERRED TO IN THE TEXT

www.authoritynutrition.com

www.boroughroseto.com/history

www.dietdoctor.com

www.drcate.com

www.fatisourfriend.com

www.fatsecret.co.uk

www.futuremedicine.com

www.gapsdiet.com

www.justgetflux.com

www.ketogenic-diet-resource.com

www.sevencountriesstudy.com

www.smashthefat.com

www.stateofobesity.org

www.webmd.com

www.westonaprice.org